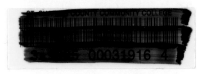

MENTAL DISCIPLINE

The Pursuit of Peak Performance

Michael K. Livingston

Human Kinetics Books
Champaign, Illinois

Library of Congress Cataloging-in-Publication Data

Livingston, Michael K., 1948—
  Mental discipline.

  Bibliography: p.
  Includes index.
  1. Sports—Psychological aspects. 2. Mind and body.
3. Mental discipline. I. Title.
GV706.4.L58 1989   796'.01   88-34807
ISBN 0-87322-228-8

Copyright © 1989 by Michael K. Livingston

ISBN: 0-87322-228-8

Developmental Editor: Kathy Kane
Production Director: Ernie Noa
Copyeditor: Bruce Owens
Assistant Editor: Robert King
Proofreader: Phaedra Hise
Typesetter: Yvonne Winsor
Text Design: Keith Blomberg
Text Layout: Jayne Clampitt and Kimberlie Henris
Cover Design: Hunter Graphics
Printed By: Braun-Brumfield

Printed in the United States of America

10 9 8 7 6 5 4 3 2 1

Human Kinetics Books
A Division of Human Kinetics Publishers, Inc.
Box 5076, Champaign, IL 61825-5076
1-800-DIAL-HKP
1-800-334-3665 (in Illinois)

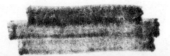

Contents

Preface

Mental Discipline: The Pursuit of Peak Performance is the culmination of my efforts to distill from my own studies and experiences certain common, fundamental strategies for learning. Throughout my life, I have been privileged to study with superb teachers—in academics, in sport, in music, and in Eastern meditative practice. I have discovered that the techniques of practice that are most effective in enhancing performance in each of these diverse pursuits are identical in certain fundamental respects. I have assembled and integrated these common essential elements of proper practice, or "right practice," into a theory of learning I have called the Theory of Right Practice.

The Theory of Right Practice is most immediately an outgrowth of my experiences as a competitor and coach in the arenas of high-level competitive athletics. My own competitive career was shaped primarily within the racing shells of Harvard University's intercollegiate rowing program, while my most extensive experiences as an athletic coach came as director of the men's intercollegiate rowing program at the University of California at Berkeley. Not only do these academic institutions possess two of the most successful and venerable rowing programs in the world, but they also enjoy well-deserved reputations as two of the world's finest intellectual centers. Not surprisingly, then, competitive athletics has involved for me a convergence of the disciplines of mind and body. I focused on this convergence in brief remarks made during an awards banquet celebrating the completion of a successful competitive rowing season at the University of California. My comments were directed to student athletes who had devoted a minimum of 3 to 4 hours per day throughout the academic year to the pursuit of peak performance in this demanding sport:

Obviously, competitive crew has been for you a discipline of the body. Your practice of crew has induced a sensitivity to and awareness of the physical body that has transformed virtually every bodily cell. You have watched your body grow and harden. You have become stronger. Your lungs and limbs are more elastic, more resilient. On a cellular level, you have facilitated and enhanced those metabolic processes that magically translate matter into propulsive energy. You have grooved neurological pathways and opened new capillaries. You have become attuned to the play of hormonal agents. You have searched for the limits of physical performance, and once you have found them you have learned to dance on their edge: on the edge of balance and imbalance, rhythm and arhythm, control and abandonment, contraction and relaxation. You have, in short, probed the untamed regions of your own physical limits. You have explored the ultimate frontier of your own living spaceship.

But crew has been far more for you than a discipline of the body. Perhaps even more emphatically, it has been a discipline of the mind. Through the daily practice, you have concentrated the mind with unwavering intensity. You have habitualized perseverance and honed the skills of disciplined commitment and focused application. Indeed, it is your will that has led you to the far reaches of your physical limits. Through the daily ritual of mindful practice, you have forged a will of steel, and then you have turned that hardened will against your physical limits whenever they have arisen; and methodically, patiently—yet relentlessly—you have pressed back those limits to reveal new worlds within your own being. And in doing so you have discovered more than the tremendous power of your body. You have discovered the power of the will. It is a power that is infinite. It is the power of belief.

Now, in *Mental Discipline: The Pursuit of Peak Performance*, I revisit these same themes, but with an ambitious and eclectic analysis that extends far beyond the realm of sport. Certainly, this analysis is intended to speak to athletes and coaches and others engaged in the pursuit of peak performance in competitive sport. Yet the concept of peak performance is not limited to athletics. Every act of mind and body potentially can be styled and gauged as a performance, and the quality of that performance invariably can be enhanced through right practice. It is my hope that this book will chart a path to peak performance within virtually any discipline of mind or body.

I have developed in these writings a firm conceptual foundation for the Theory of Right Practice. This foundation consists of a scientific and philosophical inquiry into the nature of the human mind. *Mental Discipline: The Pursuit of Peak Performance* explores the scientific disciplines of exercise physiology, neurophysiology, and quantum physics, together with the Eastern disciplines of meditative introspection, to develop a model of human consciousness that is grounded in the extraordinary power of the individual will. It is the mastery of the willpower of the mind that provides the indispensable foundation for right practice. I offer *Mental Discipline: The Pursuit of Peak Performance* as a guidebook on the path to a mastery of the will.

Acknowledgments

I would like to thank those who, through their own systems of "right practice," have developed the general fund of knowledge on which I have drawn in the preparation of this book. In particular, I wish to thank all those who have permitted me to reproduce copyrighted material, not only for the use of the material but also for the benefit of their insights and analyses. I also wish to thank Bob Carland for his skillful redrawing of the figures.

I am deeply grateful to the many superb teachers who have guided me in cultivating disciplines of both mind and body. I wish to thank especially John C. and Ethel M. Livingston, Arlynna Howell Livingston, Emily Rulison Smith, Harry L. Parker, and Lama Thubten Yeshe.

Finally, I wish to thank Rainer Martens and the editorial staff of Human Kinetics Books, especially Kathryn Kane and Joanne Fetzner.

1

The Paths to Knowledge

For me there is only the traveling on paths that have heart, on any path that may have heart. There I travel, and the only worthwhile challenge is to traverse its full length. And there I travel, looking, looking, breathlessly.

Don Juan, Carlos Castaneda

Perhaps the most obvious distinction between the human species and most other forms of life is that we are better learners. To be sure, we still stumble into much of our learning, but we also have developed sophisticated systems of learning. This book describes one such system.

The system of learning presented here is based on the concept of practice. Indeed, the entire system can be encapsulated in the maxim that "practice makes perfect." If this emphasis disappoints and discourages readers seeking a quick and easy path to skill or knowledge, so be it. The fact is that to reach the summit, one must climb the mountain. There are, of course, many paths up the mountain. Some paths are more difficult than others. Some are more circuitous than others. Some paths never reach the summit at all. But it is certain that one who does not climb will not reach the top.

Practice involves systematic thought or conduct performed for the purpose of acquiring knowledge or skills. The essential aspect of practice is its implication of *purposeful* thought or conduct. It is the concept of purpose that distinguishes practice from experience. Without question, it is

1

possible to learn from virtually any experience. Mere experience, however, is a clumsy and limited way to learn, and it certainly does not constitute practice. Only when experience is systematized by the application of purpose does it rise to the level of practice. Although practice may make perfect, then, it is purpose that makes practice.

The extreme generality of the aphorism that ''practice makes perfect'' renders it practically meaningless. Beneath the gloss of this self-evident apothegm lies a complex inquiry into the nature of perfect practice. It is this inquiry that occupies the pages of this book. I develop and present here a system of *Right Practice*, in which the efficacy of practice is maximized in the pursuit of perfection.

Everyday notions of practice focus primarily on skill development. Practice, in other words, commonly suggests repeated performance of some physical act for the purpose of developing skill or proficiency in that act. The notion of practice, therefore, is commonly perceived to apply principally to physical training. As a consequence, the mental aspect to practice frequently is neglected. Such neglect constitutes the most common and serious error of practice. Rote, mindless repetition is not practice.

The concept of purpose, then, lies at the heart of Right Practice. Purpose brings to practice a profound mental dimension. It is purpose that focuses the practice, and it is the intensity and specificity of that focus that governs the efficacy of the practice. The role of purpose in focusing practice is intricate and subtle, but its importance cannot be overemphasized.

The purpose that focuses the practice is a creation of mind. Right Practice, therefore, is mindful practice. It is from this basic truth that this book departs, and it is to this same basic truth that it eventually will return. Even techniques of practice designed specifically to teach or enhance a complex motor skill must be anchored in mindfulness. It is, ultimately, the mind that teaches the body. The focus of practice must be first and foremost within and on the mind, for only then can the mind focus the practices of the body.

In short, the mind must be the preeminent focus of Right Practice. And just as the body is trained by a system of practice, so too must the mind be trained through practice. Right Practice that trains the processes of mind constitutes a *discipline of mind*.

These are, of course, writings—letters and words, then sentences, paragraphs, and chapters. But fundamentally, these are words—many words. Each word is a concept, symbolizing a specific state of conceptual awareness. The relationships of states of conceptual awareness to one another over time make up the processes of mind. A practice that seeks to train the processes of mind is a discipline of mind. These words constitute such a discipline of mind.

Words have materiality. They exist in time and space, either as objective symbols on a page or as sound waves, originating in the physiological processes of speech. Yet words also have a conceptual essence that is incorporeal. This essence, which consists of the abstract idea that gives the word symbol meaning, cannot be located in time and space. It has no length, width, or depth. It has no odor, taste, color, feel, or sound. It is invisible. It is a pure experience of mind.

Mind is an extremely provocative word. It distinguishes itself from the material universe, including the physical body. It declares itself indispensable to Right Practice.

Mind and Matter: East and West

> *The most beautiful and most profound emotion we can experience is the sensation of the mystical. It is the sower of all true science. He to whom this emotion is a stranger, who can no longer wonder and stand rapt in awe, is as good as dead. To know that what is impenetrable to us really exists, manifesting itself as the highest wisdom and the most radiant beauty which our dull faculties can comprehend only in their most primitive forms—this knowledge, this feeling is at the center of true religiousness.*
>
> Albert Einstein

This distinction between the immaterial mind and the corporeal universe strikes to the heart of all philosophical traditions. The mind contains all subjective awareness of an objective, material universe. And yet the mind seems entirely contained by a physical body—and more precisely, by a brain—which belongs to that objective material universe.

Are there, then, two distinct levels to reality—one of corporeal things and another of incorporeal mind? Or do the two apparent levels of reality merge in some way? These questions are pivotal to the design of a Theory of Right Practice.

There are two opposing approaches to these questions, and they represent the major philosophical and cultural orientations now dominating human awareness. The approaches are from East and West. These words of direction imply respective points of geographical and cultural origin. And although this simplistic, popular distinction between a Western and an Eastern approach to knowledge is somewhat contrived and labored, it is fundamentally not without profound substance. It is a distinction employed incautiously in this book in reference to the antithetical conceptual paradigms of objectivism and subjectivism.

The approach from the West is grounded in the objectivism and empiricism of the scientific method. The Western path to knowledge is predicated on the presumption that all creation consists of organizations of matter and energy in space and time. All phenomena—including, ultimately, phenomena of mind—are presumed to possess some objective material foundation. The faith of Western positivism is that there is an ordered form to the phenomenal universe and that the laws governing that order are revealed through objective observations and empirical measurements of the patterns of relationship between matter and energy in space and time.

Such observations and measurements require that all creation be differentiated into distinguishable and measurable objects and events in space and time. These discrete objects and events are ordered with respect to one another through the inference of causal energies or forces that themselves lack corporeality but that exist and are revealed only through their effects on material objects. Energy cannot exist apart from matter, and matter cannot exist apart from energy. Together, energy and matter constitute a universe of physical phenomena, manifest in time and space, that exhibits discernible patterns of relationship between discrete material objects.

These patterns of relationship are presumed to give rise to the unimaginably complex organization of systems of matter and energy that constitute individual sentient beings and even to the subjective experience of conscious awareness. The Western approach to knowledge, in other words, begins with the perception of patterns of relationship in space and time between discrete corporeal objects and leads ultimately to the mind itself.

The way of the East begins within the mind. The first and preeminent reality for the Eastern approach to knowledge is subjective awareness, which lacks the corporeality that comprised the rudiment of Western positivism. This subjectivism of the East supplants the objectivism and empiricism of Western science with highly evolved systems of introspection. Physical phenomena are understood to exist as a function of mind and need not meet objective tests of materiality. Objects exist if they are discernible within subjective awareness, whether or not they are distinguishable and measurable within an objective space and time. The mind, ultimately, is the sole faculty of perception through which all creation is realized.

The way of the East consequently conceives of the individual physical body, including the brain, as a projection of the mind. Indeed, even the terms of corporeality and the laws of relationship imposing order on a material universe are ultimately conceived as projections of mind. All creation, therefore, is contained within the mind and is accessible through sophisticated and rigorous techniques of introspection.

The approach of the East has an alluring self-evidence that is recognized within the West. There is simply no escape from the recognition that subjective awareness necessarily accompanies all perception and cognition. This understanding is reflected in René Descartes' familiar postulate: *cogito ergo sum*—"I think, therefore I am." But as the West has become increasingly committed to the positivism and empiricism of an objective scientific methodology, that postulate has been inverted: "I am, therefore I think."

Ultimately, neither West nor East requires that a definitive distinction be made between body and mind. Being and thinking are too intimately joined to permit the existence of one without the other. Still, the Eastern approach to perception conceives of the body as a function of mind, whereas the way of the West conceives of the mind as a function of body. The Eastern approach to knowledge examines the processes of mind to discern the laws of consciousness presumed to govern all creation. The Western approach to knowledge examines the processes of matter and energy to discern laws of mechanistic determinism presumed to govern all creation. A discipline of mind must accommodate both the laws of objective determinism and the laws of subjective consciousness.

The way of the West has extended the processes of mind into the farthest reaches of the physical universe, extracting highly sophisticated laws of mechanistic determinism. These systems of knowledge concerning the material universe are incredibly powerful and compelling. They permit the prediction of both galactic and subatomic phenomena with extreme accuracy. They are both highest wisdom and common sense. They form the basis for virtually all aspects of technological civilization. And ultimately, the laws of mechanistic determinism are conceived not only to govern the relationship between corporeal objects within the phenomenal universe—including the organization of matter and energy constituting the physical body and its functional systems—but also to give rise to the processes of mind.

In Pursuit of Right Practice

Reason enslaves all whose minds are not strong enough to master her.

George Bernard Shaw

Because the way of the East begins with subjective awareness, the design of an Eastern system of practice for training the processes of mind need not be justified and rationalized in objective, empirical terms. Such concepts as "purpose," "volition," "attention," and "will" all possess an irrefutable subjective meaning. Even the existence and operation of the mind itself, as a proper focus for a system of practice, is subjectively self-evident. Not surprisingly, therefore, a number of sophisticated and powerful disciplines of mind have evolved within the East based on techniques of meditative introspection.

The West, of course, is not without its own systems of introspection and practices of mind. Yet these systems generally lack the purity of design that characterizes the more highly evolved disciplines of mind spawned within the introspective traditions of the East. In fact, many of the putative disciplines of mind that have proliferated recently within the West, whether styled as religious practice or self-improvement practice, are Westernized adaptations of Eastern traditions.

To be sure, many Western systems of mental training employ techniques of unquestionable efficacy, and the more sophisticated systems have woven these techniques into internally cohesive and consistent conceptual paradigms. Such conceptual systems arise in a multiplicity of forms. Esoteric systems of mental practice have evolved within the monastic orders of certain Western religions as well as within Western stylings of Eastern religious disciplines. In addition, a wide variety of secular conceptual paradigms embodying systems of mental practice have evolved.

The Westernized presentations of techniques of mental practice generally are not grounded in the bedrock subjectivist faith of the East. Many even claim to be anchored in the objectivism and empiricism of the West. The claim to a foundation in objective truth is not made idly. There is within the West a certain skepticism with regard to theories and ideas that do not lay claim to conceptual roots in objectivism. The subjectivist "faith," in other words, is understood to be a lesser truth than the empirical measurements and "proofs" of objectivism.

The West, then, is prone to look with condescension on the Eastern traditions of introspection. Meanwhile, it pursues its own disciplines ostensibly grounded in empirical fact rather than introspective faith. This book follows that pursuit to its end. And ultimately, it is found to be a dead end.

The Western path to knowledge is explored in considerable detail in chapters 2 through 7. It is traced from the peripheral energy and contractile systems implicated in physical training, through the neuronal pathways that mediate and control these systems, to the executive control center localized in the brain. And there, within the brain, the search for the mind begins in earnest. That search leads ever deeper into the physiological mechanisms of the brain, from the cellular domain to the molecular domain and even to the atomic and subatomic domains. Finally, deep within the subatomic "quantum" domain, the quest for an objective, empirical model of the phenomenal universe simply ends. And this end comes, unfortunately, before the Western path to knowledge has reached the mind.

Ultimately, the positivism of the West is found to be inextricably bound to a system of cognition presumptively involving deterministic interactions of matter and energy in time and space. There is no room in such a system of cognition for original acts of mind. The force or power of the mind, which in these writings is termed the *will*, can no more escape the ubiquitous forces of determinism than can any other element of the phenomenal universe. Unlike the subjectivist faith of the East, the objectivism of the West cannot on its terms accommodate the notion of mind as an original causal force. Put simply, there is no place for individual free will on the Western path to knowledge. This is not an easy proposition to accept, and these writings explore in some detail the frontier between the incorporeal mind and the corporeal universe in an effort to elucidate this critical point.

So what is the value of enduring the sometimes tortuous and labyrinthine path of the West, when the signposts at the outset warn that it is a dead end? There are two answers to this important threshold question. First, it is imperative that the limitations of the objectivism and empiricism of the West be understood and that their significance be appreciated. A system of knowledge that lays claim to objective truth cannot be assailed by subjective faith alone. If such a system is vulnerable, it is vulnerable only on its own terms of cognition. The Western system of knowledge must be turned against itself. It is not enough, in other words, to stand aside from the Western path to knowledge and simply declare as an act of faith that it is ultimately limited. Instead, one must walk the path fully, for only by traversing its length and arriving at its end will the limits of the path be known with certainty. And it is this certainty that forms the fertile field in which the seeds of Right Practice must be sown.

This certainty, which lies at the threshold of a Theory of Right Practice, involves the recognition that the verities of the West are no less articles of faith than are the verities of the East. It is, in essence, a question of first principles. The faith of the East, premised on an internal, incorporeal reality of subjective awareness, easily accommodates the willpower of the mind. The faith of the West, anchored to an external, corporeal reality of objective determinism, has no place for the freedom of the human will. Yet the nonexistence of the will is no more proved by its exclusion from the objective reality of the West than its existence is established by its inclusion within the subjective reality of the East. Indeed, the concept of "proof" must be understood on this deeper level of analysis to be indistinguishable from faith. The certainty required by Right Practice, then, involves a recognition that there is at the heart of learning an unavoidable *choice of faiths*. It is not a choice between subjective faith and objective truth. It is simply a choice of faiths. To understand this with certainty is absolutely necessary if the choice of will is to be made with sufficient confidence and commitment.

The choice of faith in the willpower of the mind does not require a wholesale rejection or abandonment of the objectivist faith of the West. It does, however, require that the objectivist faith of the West be confined within its proper boundaries. And this requirement embodies the second reason that it is essential to explore fully the realm of objective determinism. The practitioner, in short, must know well the limitations of objectivism.

The willpower of the mind is not everywhere and always accessible. In fact, the mind also contains the objectivism of the West, which is grounded on the proposition that the phenomenal universe is governed by strict laws of mechanistic determinism. It is only at the boundaries of this deterministic universe that the force of will is accessible. The frontiers of the deterministic universe therefore must become familiar to those who would gain access to the willpower of the mind. An exploration of the deterministic universe reveals that it is limited both in time and in space. It is at these limits of time and space that the force of will becomes accessible.

These writings present a theory and system of learning based on Right Practice, which involves the purposeful exercise of the willpower of the mind. The system of practice that trains the will is a *discipline of mind*. The power of the will is not a force of logic or intellect but is a force of faith and belief. It is a power that is accessible only at the temporal and spatial boundaries of the deterministic universe. Right Practice therefore requires that the mind systematically reach to the limits of the deterministic universe, where the force of will becomes accessible. The will power of the mind then can be recruited to define and pursue the purpose that focuses the practice.

An Overview: Toward a Discipline of Mind

We are perceivers. . . . The world that we perceive, though, is an illusion. It was created by a description that was told to us since the moment that we were born.

We, the luminous beings, are born with two rings of power, but we use only one to create the world. That ring, which is hooked very soon after we are born, is reason, and its companion is talking. Between the two they concoct and maintain the world.

So, in essence, the world that your reason wants to sustain is the world created by a description and its dogmatic and inviolable rules, which the reason learns to accept and defend.

The secret of the luminous beings is that they have another ring of power which is never used, the will. The trick of the sorcerer is the same trick of the average man. Both have a description; one, the average man, upholds it with his reason; the other, the sorcerer, upholds it with his will. Both descriptions have their rules and the rules are perceivable, but the advantage of the sorcerer is that will is more engulfing than reason.

Don Juan, Carlos Castaneda

This is not an easy book to read and understand. It is neither anecdotal nor prescriptive. In its attempt to develop a comprehensive and useful theory of learning, the book plunges deeply into both scientific information and philosophical analysis. The disciplines of science and philosophy are, of course, intimately linked. In fact, it is an implicit theme of this book that, in any ultimate or absolute sense, they are indistinguishable.

There are, then, two fundamental dimensions to these writings. First, the foundation of this book consists of an analytical inquiry into the mechanisms and processes involved in learning. This inquiry begins with an investigation of the physiological processes implicated in physical training, leading to the postulation of *the principle of Right Practice*. Next, the book embarks on a rigorous but selective exposition and analysis of neurophysiology and theoretical physics in an attempt to fathom the deep processes underlying the phenomenon of mind. The book concludes that any "ultimate" understanding of the nature of mind is destined to rest on acts of subjective faith rather than on indestructible pillars of objective, empirical "proof." Accordingly, the philosophical construct presented in this book combines a subjective faith in the freedom of the individual will with the objective "proofs" of neurophysiology and theoretical physics to derive a synthesized Conceptual Model of Mind, which is grounded on two fundamental postulates: *the principle of conceptual awareness* and *the principle of indeterminacy*.

The second dimension to this book consists of the development of a comprehensive, eclectic theory of learning called the Theory of Right Practice. This theory is developed through the application of the principle of Right Practice (embodied within the Physiological Model of Physical Training) to the principle of conceptual awareness and the principle of indeterminacy (embodied within the Conceptual Model of Mind). In the contemplation of the Theory of Right Practice, the willpower of the mind is understood to be accessible to modulate the forces of determinism, which otherwise would be absolutely controlling. Right Practice therefore is conceived to involve the purposeful exercise of the willpower of the mind. The system of practice that trains the will involves a discipline of mind. The Theory of Right Practice provides a systematic exposition of the path to such a discipline of mind.

It should be clear from this introduction that the philosophical treatise that is at the heart of this book cannot be separated from the scientific analysis on which it is grounded. To the extent possible, however, I have attempted to make both the philosophy and the science accessible to the layreader. The Theory of Right Practice emerges from these pages piece by piece, as if it is an immense and complex puzzle. The puzzle unquestionably is challenging, but all of the necessary pieces are provided and their interrelationships explained. And once the puzzle is assembled and whole, it becomes clear that it exceeds and transcends the sum of its parts.

Here, then, is the sequence of analysis contained in these writings, leading ultimately to a convergence of West and East in a unified Theory of Right Practice: In chapter 2, high-level athletic training is analyzed in order to extrapolate a Physiological Model of Physical Training. This model is conceived to embody the *principle of Right Practice*, together with two subsidiary rules of operation: *the rule of specificity of practice* and *the rule of intensity of practice*. Chapter 3 contains a relatively sophisticated exposition of the physiological processes implicated in physical training.

In chapter 4, the cellular and molecular processes integral to the conduction of neuronal impulses within the central nervous system are analyzed in an attempt to determine the physiological bases for sensory reception, motor response, conceptual memory, and conscious awareness. This analysis is then extrapolated into an encompassing Physiological Model of Mind, in which specific states of conceptual awareness are modeled as the immaterial subjective experiences attendant on specific states of electrochemical brain activity. Awareness, perceived to arise as either volition or attention—and always as a conceptualization involving delimitations of matter and energy in space and time—is understood to be a precise reflection of the binary physiological processes with which it is inescapably partnered. Chapter 5 contains a relatively technical explication of the principal physiological processes of the brain on which the Physiological Model of Mind is grounded.

The atomic and subatomic processes underlying physical reality are analyzed in chapter 6 in order to identify the fundamental laws governing the phenomenal universe, including the universe of the human brain. An analysis of contemporary evidence and theory with respect to these most fundamental and elementary processes reveals inescapable limitations on human cognition of an external physical reality. Not only is there found to be no way to accommodate the willpower of the mind within contemporary theoretical physics, but the Empirical Model of the Phenomenal Universe itself is found to be unavoidably limited. Chapter 7 contains an extremely selective but relatively technical exposition of the historical development and present status of certain fundamental themes within the discipline of theoretical physics.

The Physiological Model of Mind and the Empirical Model of the Phenomenal Universe embody a strictly deterministic conception of physical reality. Conceptual awareness, in the contemplation of the Physiological Model of Mind, is styled as an incorporeal epiphenomenon that is strictly determined by attendant physical processes but that has no direct causal effect on the physical universe. The Physiological Model of Mind and the Empirical Model of the Phenomenal Universe therefore do not provide the necessary philosophical foundation for the Theory of Right Practice. Consequently, a Conceptual Model of Mind is hypothesized in chapter 8 to provide the indispensable foundation for a Theory of Right Practice based on the willpower of the mind. This model is supported by two fundamental postulates: *the principle of conceptual awareness* and *the principle of indeterminacy*. Informing the principle of conceptual awareness are *the rule of relative properties, the rule of equal opposition, the rule of limits*, and *the rule of failure*. Informing the principle of indeterminacy are *the rule of determinism* and *the rule of will*. These two principles, in combination with the principle of Right Practice—and together with the rules that govern their operation—comprise the precepts of the Theory of Right Practice. Chapter 9 contains a brief description of two consummate systems of mental practice that have evolved within the East: the Buddhist practices of *Vipassana* meditation and the Hindu practices of *yoga*.

In chapter 10 the application of the principle of Right Practice to the principle of conceptual awareness and the principle of indeterminacy gives rise to the Theory of Right Practice. The willpower of the mind is the sole instrument of practice, and Right Practice involves the use of the will to focus awareness in the present moment, as either volition or attention, in pursuit of failure. Failure manifests as a performance gap between the performance mandated by the forces of determinism and an image of purpose conceived through the force of will. Because all acts of body and mind manifest preeminently as conceptual awareness, failure arises as a conceptual gap between a particular chain of conceptual awareness and a conceptual image of purpose. Right Practice involves the attempt to bridge the conceptual gap through the application of the force of will, with maximum specificity and intensity, in the present moment of conceptual awareness. Chapter 11 contains an application of the Theory of Right Practice to athletic training (competitive rowing), musical training (the violin), and intellectual training (creative thought).

2

A Physiological Model of Physical Training: The Theory

At the peak of tremendous and victorious effort, while the blood is pounding in your head, all suddenly becomes quiet within you. Everything seems clearer and whiter than ever before, as if great spotlights had been turned on. At that moment you have the conviction that you contain all the power in the world, that you are capable of everything, that you have wings. There is no more precious moment in life than this, the white moment, and you will work very hard for years just to taste it again.

Yuri Vlasov, Soviet weightlifter

I have identified the concept of purpose as integral and indispensable to Right Practice and have posited purpose, in turn, as a creation of mind. The mind, in other words, is understood to focus the practices of the body through the application of purpose.

Purpose, conceived in this way, becomes a state of mind. The Theory of Right Practice is based on the proposition that such states of mind have associated *force fields*. The force field of the mind is called *willpower*, or simply the will, and it is conceived as a causal force able to act on the physical body. The physical body, of course, consists of all the constituent organic systems, including the brain and central nervous system. Right Practice therefore involves transforming a state of mind into a state of body through the agency of the will. The organizing principle of the mind is purpose or, more precisely, a conceptual *image of purpose*. The organizing force is the will. The state of mind, focused as an image of purpose, acts as an archetype for the creation, by the force of the will, of a corresponding state of body.

There is, of course, a profound conceptual gap between a state of mind and a corresponding state of body. As discussed in chapter 1, the mind is incorporeal and abstract, whereas the body (including the brain) is understood to be definite and corporeal. An image of purpose, as a state of mind, has no discernible or measurable existence in time and space. It is simply a state of subjective awareness. States of body, on the other hand, are comprehensible entirely in terms of the interactions of detectable and measurable forces and objects within an objective phenomenal universe of time and space. Two parallel realms of cognition therefore arise in consciousness: the subjective realm of the mind governed by the force of will and the objective realm of the corporeal phenomenal universe governed by the forces of mechanistic determinism.

The concept of practice introduced in chapter 1 presumes that the will-power of the mind is able to exert a causal force within the objective, corporeal realm of determinism. This proposition is profoundly unsettling to the determinist, for the introduction of an alien undetermined or "free" force into a closed, deterministic universe nullifies its supposed determinism. The deterministic perspective trivializes the force of the will into insignificance, either by conceiving it to be determined, or by separating it to a realm with no causal nexus to the realm of determinism.

There is, however, a middle ground between these seemingly antithetical realms of free will and determinism. It is a middle ground in which the forces of will and determinism are conceived to interact, and it is located on the border separating the deterministic realm of time and space from the realm of pure mind. The transmutation of a state of mind into a correlative state of body, which is the hypothesized essence of Right Practice, occurs within this border zone. The force field emanating from the image of purpose enters the practice as the willpower of the mind. It does not, however, act there alone. The states of the physical body also arise as manifestations of the forces of determinism. In fact, the forces of determinism predominate in shaping the states of body, as the laws of mechanistic determinism largely dictate the progression of body states from one point in space and time to the next.

It is only through the application of the willpower of the mind, emanating as a force field from a purposeful state of mind, that the otherwise irresistible currents of determinism can be modulated. And the forces of determinism are modulated by the force of will only within the border zone that lies outside the deterministic realm of time and space. States of body therefore are not ordained purely by acts of will; rather, the will acts together with the forces of determinism to shape and "synthesize" a state of body. The willpower of the mind, in other words, acts on the forces of determinism to "co"-"ordinate" a state of body in the image of a corresponding state of mind.

This "coordination" is clearly reflected in those states of body involved in the performance of complex motor skills and especially in the consummate performances of high-level athletics. In fact, the idea of coordination is commonly understood to encompass virtually all aspects of complex motor performances. The concepts customarily associated with motor skills—such as strength, power, speed, endurance, balance, and grace—are comfortably subsumed within the concept of coordination. And athletics, in essence, is both a celebration and a test of the majesty and mystery of coordination.

It is axiomatic that Right Practice is reflected in high achievement. Through an analysis of high achievement, it is therefore presumed possible to identify the primary characteristics of Right Practice. Sophisticated mechanisms have been developed for measuring and evaluating performances of the body. These measurement processes and evaluation standards are perhaps most highly refined within the realm of competitive athletics, where discrete physical skills are tested, measured, and evaluated. Consequently, high achievement within competitive athletics is readily identifiable, and the techniques of physical training that produce high achievement are accessible to analysis.

Athletics, particularly at its highest levels, is a realm of intensely subjective inquiry and enterprise in which each participant attempts to distill general training and performance principles from the fires of personal experience. Generalized rules of practice have evolved over time, reflecting a compounding of such subjective experience. And subjective evaluations of the efficacy of various training regimens routinely have been tested in the arenas of competition, frequently against objective standards such as time and distance. Until recently, however, the immense number of potential variables in training and performance have made athletics somewhat resistant to a scientific methodology based on objective quantification and experimental verification.

The analytical powers of science have now been turned on the realm of athletics. Scientists of varied specialties have begun to explore the realm of athletics, thus rapidly expanding the scientific understanding of physical training. This thrust of scientific empiricism into the realm of competitive athletics has substantially confirmed the efficacy of the systems of practice that already had evolved. In the process, many of the physiological mechanisms of learning that underlie these systems of training have been identified and analyzed. And ultimately, this scientific understanding of the physiology of physical training has been turned back on these systems of practice in order to refine the techniques of training and enhance the training benefit.

This unique synthesis of introspection and empiricism within athletics yields a powerful Physiological Model of Physical Training. This model identifies the organic processes of the body involved in particular complex motor skills and demonstrates how these processes are enhanced through practice. The model is a first step on the path to an understanding of how a purposeful state of mind can modulate the forces of determinism to coordinate a particular state of body.[1]

The Physiological Subsystems of Motor Performance

But strength is more than the transformation of matter into other forms of matter, it is the transformation of the whole cycle of air and light into matter and back again. In fact, it completes Einstein's equation of matter and energy and translates it into the human, the living incarnation.

Yehudi Menuhin

At the outset, it is important to recognize that there are two fundamental dimensions to the focus of mind in an image of purpose. As previously suggested, coordination involves the application of the force of will to forge a state of body that approaches congruency with a corresponding state of mind embodied in an image of purpose. Simply put, the state of mind coordinates the state of body. This aspect of coordination is a reflection of a *hard-focused* image of purpose with an associated force field that is projective and efferent in its operation. Such an outwardly directed image of purpose arises as *volition*.

The second dimension to the focus of an image of purpose is more subtle but no less significant. It involves the application of the force of will to create a state of mind corresponding to a particular state of body. The image of purpose gives rise to a receptive field that attracts and responds to input from a specific genre of body states. In other words, the state of mind opens itself to be coordinated by a particular state of body. This aspect of coordination is a reflection of a *soft-focused* image of purpose with an associated force field that is receptive and afferent in its operation, and it is termed *attention*.

Any complex motor performance will involve both aspects of coordination. Both the hard focus of volition and the soft focus of attention are critical to the effective transposition of a purposeful state of mind to a coordinated state of body. Volition and attention are, then, the two correlative focuses to the willpower of the mind.

The force of will, focused in either its projective mode as volition or its receptive mode as attention, potentially can coordinate a state of the body in terms of an image of purpose. The organizing principle (i.e., the image of purpose) and its coordinating force field (i.e., the willpower of mind) therefore are conceived to have the capacity to control the body's contractile system and to coordinate a particular complex motor performance. It bears reiteration, however, that this control is far from absolute. The formulation of a particular image of purpose does not automatically guarantee that a corresponding state of body will manifest. For example, an image of purpose that conceives the body as flying, no matter how specific and intense, will not result in a flying body. There are, in other words, certain physiological constraints on the causal potency of the force of will. These constraints are a reflection of the powerful forces of determinism as modulated over time by the force of the will. This modulation effect, then, is the essence of physical training.

A Physiological Model of Physical Training must accommodate such adaptations and enhancements to the physiological systems that generate, control, and constrain complex motor performances. And, as previously suggested, the physiological systems most proximately implicated in the performance of complex motor skills are components of the body's contractile system. The contractile system, therefore, is the initial focus of analysis in the derivation of a Physiological Model of Physical Training.

The contractile system is by no means monolithic but is composed of numerous distinguishable "subsystems." There are, in fact, a vast multitude of functional subsystems that are coordinated to achieve each complex motor performance. These subsystems are not only linked sequentially to accomplish a compound motor task but are also layered on multiple levels. The layering begins on a gross, macroscopic level and descends into increasingly specific microscopic and submicroscopic levels. In these writings, an approximate and relatively arbitrary distinction is drawn between the higher-level, more general functional subsystems, which are termed "macrosystems," and the deeper-level, more specific functional subsystems, which are termed "microsystems." As a rough approximation, the levels of layering can be conceived as follows: the organism level, the organ level, the cellular level, the molecular level, the atomic level, the subatomic level, and the conceptual level. The organism and organ levels are considered macrosystemic in nature, whereas the cellular, molecular, atomic, and subatomic levels are categorized as microsystemic domains. The conceptual level exists only on the incorporeal level of pure mind.

A complex motor performance involves the coordination of integral macrosystems and microsystems on all levels simultaneously. The image of purpose that forms the template for coordination of the motor activity (and that resides on the conceptual level) obviously does not specifically and simultaneously contemplate the coordination of every constituent microsystem implicated in that motor performance. Generally, the image of purpose conceives of a complex motor performance on one of the higher levels of macrosystemic function. For example, many images of purpose are task specific, contemplating a particular motor performance on the "organism" macrosystemic level, in terms of the coordinated gross motions of the entire body. This, in fact, is the common notion of coordination. And for ordinary purposes and ordinary motor performances, such a nonspecific, macrosystemic image of purpose may be sufficient. Yet it has now become clear that the forces of coordination are more effectively applied at the deeper levels of microsystemic function. The practice, in other words, becomes more effective when the image of purpose is focused with greater specificity, and this requires that the focus be trained on some deeper functional microsystem.

The appreciation of the importance of specificity in physical training is a reflection of the critical role of failure in the process of learning complex motor skills. When particular motor skills are conceptualized as a task-specific image of purpose on the highest macrosystemic level, failure is simply the inability to accomplish the task. Repetitive practice of the implicated motor skills is commonly understood to enhance the likelihood that the task eventually will be achieved. In fact, repetitive attempts to achieve a particular complex motor skill are universally understood to be an effective strategy to learn that motor skill. It is hardly a profound revelation, therefore, that failed attempts to achieve an image of purpose are the path to eventual success and achievement.

This basic, instinctive approach to motor learning has of course been refined and perfected within the framework of competitive athletics. The underlying notion that "practice makes perfect" has not really changed significantly, but the nature of practice has changed. Practitioners have come to understand that the more precisely and intensely their practice is focused, the more rapidly they learn. And most significantly, they have learned that the focus must be on the specific microsystem that is subject to failure and that the training regimen must stress that microsystem to failure. In other words, the efficacy of the practice has been recognized to depend on the specificity and intensity with which the practice targets the failure of a limiting constituent microsystem.

The Parameters of Failure

> One never knows what is enough until one knows what is more than enough.
>
> William Blake

Failures in a motor performance are, from the highest-level macrosystemic perspective, failures of the contractile system. Yet such failures are manifested in a variety of forms that are susceptible to categorization. In rough terms, failures within the contractile macrosystem can be classified as failures of coordination, failures of strength, failures of power, and failures of endurance. These four genres of failure are reflections of the four predominant parameters of performance: coordination, strength, power, and endurance.

The concept of coordination already has been invoked, of course, as the process mediating a particular state of mind and a corresponding state of body. As such, it incorporates all aspects and parameters of performance, including strength, power, and endurance. As a performance parameter itself, however, coordination refers to the integration of discrete states of body rather than the integration of mind and body. It involves, in other words, the coordination of the constituent subsystems of the contractile system. Eventually, it will become clear that, even as a performance parameter, coordination governs the subsidiary performance parameters of strength, power, and endurance. Yet failures of the contractile system are experienced not only as failures of coordination but also (and distinctively) as failures of these three subsidiary performance parameters.

It is important to understand the distinction between the performance parameters of strength, power, and endurance. Strength refers to the amount of force that can be generated in one voluntary maximum muscle contraction either isometrically or through a specific range of contraction. The maintenance or repetition of that single maximum contraction implicates factors relating to muscle endurance and compromises strength. The concept of strength is purely a measurement of force irrespective of the velocity of the contraction. Power, on the other hand, is a measure of both the force and the speed of one voluntary muscle contraction through a specific range of contraction. Power involves, therefore, the correlation of the strength of a given muscle contraction with the velocity of that contraction. It is a measure of the amount of force per unit time that can be generated by a single muscle contraction. Generally, as the velocity of a contraction increases, fewer muscle fibers can be mobilized to power the contraction, and strength consequently is diminished. Similarly, the speed of a contraction generally will increase as resistance decreases, given an invariant application of force. Muscular endurance, finally, is a measure of the length of time a given level of power can be maintained.

The importance of any particular performance parameter to a given motor skill obviously will depend on the degree to which that performance parameter is implicated in the motor skill. More precisely, a particular performance parameter becomes significant for the purposes of physical training only when it is identified as an actual or potential point of failure in the coordinated motor performance. When a specific performance parameter is recognized to be vulnerable to failure, that precise parameter properly is targeted for practice. The focus may be on coordination, strength, power, or endurance. Practice time and energy, which always are limited, therefore can be economically trained on the weakest links in the chain of coordinated motor response, and learning occurs where it is most needed.

The failure of a particular parameter of performance involves the failure of a specific physiological macrosystem that is integral to that performance parameter. Although virtually all performance failures will manifest ultimately as failures of the contractile system, the underlying source of failure will reside in any of three primary macrosystems: the contractile macrosystem, the energy macrosystem, or the neuronal macrosystem. Significantly, the failure of a particular macrosystem will be experienced as a failure of a corresponding performance parameter. A failure of endurance will involve failure within the energy macrosystem. A failure of strength or power will involve failure within the contractile macrosystem. And a failure of coordination will involve failure in the neuronal macrosystem. Failure means either the cessation of appropriate function or the inability to achieve appropriate function. By focusing the practice on the failures of a given performance parameter, then, the practice is focused on the failure of a specific functional macrosystem. Yet the specificity of focus does not end with these three macrosystems.

The contractile macrosystem involves a multiplicity of physiological microsystems that coordinate to cause a shortening, or contraction, of a particular muscle fiber. The recruitment of a particular muscle fiber for contraction, however, is a function of the neuronal macrosystem. The neuronal macrosystem also consists of a vast array of constituent physiological microsystems that coordinate to transmit neuronal impulses to the contractile microsystems within a particular muscle fiber, thereby triggering or inhibiting contraction. And finally, the contraction of a muscle fiber necessarily implicates the energy macrosystem, which is recruited to supply the fuel necessary to energize the contractile and neuronal microsystems. The energy macrosystem is composed of numerous functional microsystems that coordinate to transmute carbohydrates, fats, and proteins into the body's fuel, adenosine triphosphate (ATP).

Many of these microsystems in the energy, contractile, and neuronal macrosystems have been analyzed by scientists on the cellular and molecular levels. A critical revelation of these analyses is that virtually all of the manifold microsystems examined evidence an enhancement of function in response to systematic stress over time. In other words, even the constituent microsystems discernible on a cellular and molecular level "improve" with practice. The functional limits of each molecular reaction integral to the recruitment and execution of a muscular contraction appear to be extended by the stress of that specific electrochemical process to its functional limits, followed by an adequate period of recovery.

The realization that underpins this focus of Right Practice on the failures of specific microsystems is that the physiological microsystems adapt positively in response to stress. Therefore, when a specific microsystem is stressed to failure and then permitted to recover, its functional limits increase. And when the functional limits of a particular microsystem are extended through practice, it becomes a stronger link in all of the physiological chains of which it is an integral component. Training is significant from a performance perspective, then, only when the microsystem that is strengthened is a "limiting," or "weak," link in a macrosystem implicated in the motor performance. For this reason, Right Practice targets the microsystems subject to failure in the particular motor performance.

Each macrosystem, then, is composed of multiple sequences and layers of functional microsystems, and it is ultimately the failure of any discrete integral microsystem that precipitates macrosystemic and performance failures. Right Practice therefore must focus on the specific limiting microsystem with an intensity sufficient to extend it to failure. With its recovery from failure, that microsystem thereafter will be a stronger link in the physiological chains that produce the desired motor performance.

Although these performance parameters and their underlying macrosystems and microsystems are conceptually distinguishable, it is important to acknowledge the ultimate integration and coordination of these functional elements into a particular complex motor performance. Viewed from a macrosystemic level, for example, the contractile system is directly controlled by the neuronal system, and the energy system is directly controlled by the contractile system. In general, a particular muscle fiber will contract only as the result of its excitation by a neuronal impulse. Moreover, the intensity of contraction by the muscle fiber is determined by the rate of transmission of neuronal impulses across the neuromuscular synapse. In other words, a specific muscle fiber is recruited to contract in support of a particular motor activity, and the intensity of its contraction is governed by the transmission of neuronal impulses to that muscle fiber. It is the intensity and duration of the muscle contraction, in turn, that determine the specific energy microsystems that will be recruited to fuel that contraction. The neuronal system, then, directly controls the contractile system and indirectly, though no less decisively, controls the energy system.

The layers and chains of microsystems, in short, are significant only by virtue of their linkage and synthesis into significant states of body. Complex motor performances are coordinated by the selection and linkage of specific combinations of these multiple microsystems, and by their sequencing over time. These processes by which the proper chains of physiological microsystems are recruited and mobilized must be enormously sophisticated in order to coordinate such complex motor activities as the performance of the Beethoven violin concerto or a 29-foot long jump. Even the motor skills involved in such mundane activities as talking and walking involve the extremely sophisticated coordination of innumerable physiological microsystems. Yet despite this elegant coordination of multiple subsystems, the fragmentation of the body into its integral physiological macrosystems and microsystems and correlative functional parameters, as a first approximation, is a convenient and powerful scheme of analysis. And eventually, that analysis will move to deeper levels from which the inadequacies and limitations of this first approximation will become apparent.

A Physiological Model of Physical Training

Monks, when one Unique Law is practiced and repeatedly done so, it leads from a sense of great terror, to great benefit, to great cessation of bondage, to great mindfulness and awareness, to acquisition of the knowledge of wisdom, to a happy life here and now, to realization of the fruits of clear vision and deliverance. What is the Unique Law? It is mindfulness of the body.

Buddha

The performance parameters of strength, power, and endurance are readily testable and quantifiable. Increments of improvement in these performance parameters resulting from particular strategies of physical training therefore are easily discernible and measurable. The performance parameter of coordination, on the other hand, is more abstract and less easily quantified. Although it is certainly possible to gauge improvements in coordination in response to physical training, such measurements are likely to be far less precise and reliable than those relating to the performance parameters of strength, power, and endurance. For this reason, the Physiological Model of Physical Training is grounded principally on an analysis of the more readily quantifiable performance parameters of strength, power, and endurance. To be sure, the Physiological Model of Physical Training that is derived from this partial analysis eventually will be applied also to the performance parameter of coordination. This application, in fact, ultimately yields the Theory of Right Practice which is the predominant theme of this book.

The Physiological Model of Physical Training is based, then, on an examination of three of the four primary performance parameters of complex motor activity: endurance, strength, and power. These performance parameters are revealed to be controlled principally by three distinguishable physiological macrosystems: the energy macrosystem, the contractile macrosystem, and the neuronal macrosystem. Within each of these three general physiological macrosystems are a vast number of constituent functional microsystems. In fact, each functional macrosystem can be conceived as a physiologically linked chain of its constituent microsystems. These linkages are both horizontal over time, reflecting the sequencing of functional microsystems, and vertical at each point in time, reflecting the layering of functional microsystems. Both the general functional macrosystem and each of its integral microsystems has a limited functional range. The functional range of the macrosystem is limited by the failure of a limiting integral microsystem. The physiological chain that constitutes the functional macrosystem is only as strong as its weakest microsystemic link. That is, each constituent microsystem implicated in the performance parameters of complex motor activity has performance limits beyond which that particular microsystem will not function. The failure of a particular microsystem will cause the failure of any functional macrosystem within which it is an integral link.

Such failures, however, have within them the seeds of success. Subjective experience and empirical analysis have revealed that when a particular microsystem is made to function at or near its performance limits through training and then is permitted to recover adequately, it gradually will undergo physiological modifications that extend those functional limits. The Physiological Model of Physical Training is premised on this understanding of the way in which the microsystems integral to the neuronal, energy, and contractile macrosystems adapt in response to the stresses of physical training.

Failures of performance therefore are a reflection of failures of some limiting constituent microsystem integral to either the contractile, the neuronal, or the energy macrosystem. It becomes clear by this analysis that failures of strength or power involve failures most proximately localized within the contractile macrosystem, and failures of endurance involve failures localized within the energy macrosystem. It also becomes clear that the precise nature of the motor performance will dictate the specific microsystems that will be functionally implicated. The failure of a particular performance parameter therefore corresponds to the failure of a specific physiological microsystem. By targeting the performance failure with maximum specificity, therefore, the limiting physiological microsystem is trained with specificity. And, of course, the underlying assumption is that by stressing that limiting microsystem to failure and then allowing it to recover, the performance limits of the microsystem are extended. This assumption is premised on both subjective experience and objective, empirical analysis, and it forms the foundation for the Physiological Model of Physical Training presented in this chapter.

The conceptual foundation for the Physiological Model of Physical Training therefore can be codified as *the principle of Right Practice*. This principle embodies the relatively self-evident notion that progress in any discipline requires Right Practice of that discipline. Right Practice, in other words, makes progress, and progress ultimately makes perfect.

The principle of Right Practice is hardly a revelatory precept. And taken alone, the principle is not particularly helpful. However, the Physiological Model of Physical Training embodies two subsidiary rules of operation that give dimension and meaning to the principle of Right Practice. These rules are *the rule of specificity of practice* and *the rule of intensity of practice*. These two operational rules define the conceptual parameters within which the practice must be focused.

The rule of specificity of practice recognizes that the efficacy of the practice is directly related to the degree of specificity with which the practice reflects the discipline. In other words, the more exactly the practice involves the specific motor skills and performance parameters that constitute the bodily discipline, the more effective the practice will be in developing that particular discipline. Indeed, the more specifically the training is able to target the precise functional microsystem that constitutes the limiting factor, or the weak link, in the macrosystemic chains integral to a particular performance failure, the more powerful will be the training effect. The practice, in short, must be focused with maximum specificity.

The rule of intensity of practice similarly recognizes that the efficacy of the practice is directly related to the intensity of the practice. Intensity is a second dimension to the focus of practice. Not only must the training regimen target the specific limiting microsystem, but it must exercise that microsystem at or near its functional limits. The degree of stress placed on the microsystem is a reflection of the intensity of the practice. Whereas the concept of specificity relates to the definition of the motor skill in the dimensions of space, the concept of intensity relates to the definition of the motor skill in the dimension of time. Specificity, in other words, refers to the external targeting of the focus of practice, whereas intensity refers to the internal power or resolution of that focus. The practice must be focused with maximum intensity within its external focus of specificity.

The principle of Right Practice therefore is based on the proposition that the specific limiting physiological microsystem should be stressed through training to failure. Yet within any system of physical training designed to enhance strength, power, or endurance, failure does not come to the practitioner as a sterile, abstract concept. Rather, it arises most frequently as a compelling sensory experience of fatigue. There are two distinguishable dimensions to this experience of fatigue. First, as discussed previously, the physiological capacities of the energy, contractile, and neuronal macrosystems involved in a given exercise are limited. Whenever the functional limits of an integral microsystemic link in an implicated macrosystemic chain are exceeded, the macrosystem fails. Yet as these physiological mechanisms are stressed toward terminal fatigue, there frequently is a concomitant stimulation of pain receptors and other negative feedback mechanisms that creates a ''mental'' specter of discomfort and distress. This mental distress constitutes the second dimension to fatigue. Both dimensions arise in concert, and the intensity of the mental component to fatigue is directly related to the proximity of the physiological mechanisms to terminal incapacity.

Exercise can terminate, therefore, either as a result of the physiological fatigue and incapacity of the energy, the neuronal, or the contractile macrosystems or as a result of the "mental" fatigue attendant on the physiological stress. Terminal fatigue of the physiological mechanisms constitutes physiological failure, whereas terminal mental fatigue is regarded, in the terminology of exercise physiologists, as "volitional" failure. The volitional failures of terminal mental fatigue cause a premature cessation of systemic function prior to physiological incapacity.

The failures of physiological incapacity are conceived to occur within the energy, contractile, and neuronal subsystems that are directly and immediately responsible for complex motor performance. Each such failure triggers positive organic adaptations within those specific microsystems that are stressed to their functional limits. Right Practice therefore has been conceived to involve the pursuit of physiological incapacity through maximum specificity and intensity of training. The specificity and intensity of the practice, in turn, are a reflection of the purpose of the practice, and purpose is a function of mind. Right Practice therefore must be mindful practice, even when the actual learning appears to transpire within peripheral functional microsystems seemingly remote from the mind. Conceptual difficulties arise, then, in discriminating between the failures of physiological systemic incapacity and the premature "volitional" failures ostensibly associated with "mental" fatigue. The escape from this potential confusion requires that "volitional failure" be understood to mean "the failure of volition." In this way, a distinction arises between Right Practice, which contemplates the pursuit of the failures of physiological incapacity through force of will (manifest alternatively as volition and attention), and nonpractice, which involves the premature failures imposed by the forces of determinism in the absence of will.

The Physiological Model of Physical Training demonstrates the paramount importance of the neuronal macrosystem in coordinating the contractile and the energy macrosystems that produce complex motor performance. Earlier in this chapter, however, states of body, including those involved in complex motor performance, were hypothesized to be potentially a function of correlative states of mind. Control over the neuronal macrosystem, then, has been linked potentially to the mind, and this control is the essence of Right Practice. The mind, in other words, has the potential to coordinate the neuronal macrosystem, which in turn coordinates the contractile and the energy macrosystems. An image of purpose has been identified as the principle of coordination, and the willpower of the mind, focused alternatively as volition and attention, has been posited as the force of coordination. Yet this skeletal conceptual framework requires substantial elaboration if it is to model the processes through which the mind exerts control over the brain and the body.

To derive such a comprehensive model, the neuronal macrosystem must be traced from the contractile and the energy macrosystems, through the peripheral neural processes, to the central nervous system, and finally to the brain. It is there, among the regulatory, sensory, and effector functions of the brain, that the mind's power of coordination appears to be localized. The path to an encompassing conceptual paradigm that accommodates this power of a state of mind to coordinate a state of brain (and therefore a state of body) must traverse the deepest recesses of the brain in search of the mind. And ultimately, that path must enter the border zone between the incorporeal realm of pure mind and the corporeal universe of time and space. It is a path through increasingly deeper layers of microsystemic function within the brain. The first level of analysis, expounded in chapters 4 and 5, explores the cellular and the molecular microsystemic layers of the brain and results in the derivation of a Physiological Model of Mind. The next level of analysis, contained in chapters 6 and 7, descends to the atomic and the subatomic microsystemic layers and yields an Empirical Model of the Phenomenal Universe. And finally, in chapter 8, the analysis crosses the boundaries of the corporeal universe and enters the realm of pure mind, culminating in a Conceptual Model of Mind, which maps the border zone beyond the corporeal, deterministic universe and describes the mechanisms and dynamics of the mind's coordination of the brain and body. This Conceptual Model of Mind provides the indispensable foundation for the Theory of Right Practice.

Note

[1]Chapter 3 contains a relatively detailed and technical exposition of the various physiological microsystems implicated in complex motor performances. In addition, chapter 3 briefly reviews the primary strategies of physical training utilized to enhance performance and summarizes many of the organic adaptations to the physiological microsystems that result from such training. The presentation contained in this chapter is substantially extrapolated from this empirical information, and the reader is therefore referred to chapter 3 for elaboration and clarification of the evidence supporting the Physiological Model of Physical Training.

3

A Physiological Model of Physical Training: The Evidence

If you want muscular strength you must exercise your muscles. If you want real will you must exercise your will. You must concentrate and refine it as a metallurgist concentrates and refines a metal. Strength exerted equals greater strength; weakness indulged equals greater weakness.

Anonymous

This chapter contains an analytical extrapolation of the Physiological Model of Physical Training. The presentation first investigates the macrosystems involved in complex movement—energy production and supply and muscle contraction—and then the techniques of practice used to enhance their performance. From these analyses, a Physiological Model of Physical Training is hypothesized. This model is then validated through a review of the major physiological adaptations that result from Right Practice.

Energy Sources

Food and oxygen are the two essential sources of fuel for the body's energy systems. Ultimately, either directly or indirectly, both derive from plants. Plants, in turn, rely on the sun to energize the systems that sustain their existence and ours.

Electromagnetic radiation from the sun is utilized by plants through the complex electrochemical processes of photosynthesis. Photosynthesis converts carbon dioxide and water into various organic molecules, releasing oxygen to the atmosphere in the process. The sun's electromagnetic energy is transformed through photosynthesis into the chemical energy that bonds carbon, hydrogen, and oxygen into particular configurations of carbohydrate molecules. This chemical energy, locked within the organic molecules of plants, may be processed through multiple layers in the food chain before becoming available to the human digestive tract, principally as carbohydrates, fats, and proteins.

Each of these classes of food—carbohydrate, fat, and protein—can be used to produce energy in the human body. Although fats yield more than twice the energy metabolized per gram than carbohydrates or proteins, carbohydrate metabolism is used most extensively during medium- to high-intensity exercise.

The digestive process reduces carbohydrates into simple sugars— glucose, fructose, and galactose—which are absorbed into the bloodstream from the gastrointestinal tract. The concentration of glucose in the bloodstream is regulated principally by the pancreatic hormone insulin. Insulin appears to increase the permeability of peripheral cell membranes to glucose, permitting increased glucose absorption from the bloodstream into body cells, including muscle cells. Blood glucose that is not utilized immediately to fuel bodily processes is converted chemically into compound chains, called glycogen, for storage principally within the muscle cells and liver. In addition, the liver converts fructose and galactose into glucose and stores excess glucose as hepatic glycogen. When more glucose is needed, the liver's store of glycogen is converted to free glucose by enzymatic action and reenters the bloodstream. This reconversion of glycogen to glucose within the liver, called glycogenolysis, is regulated through the pancreatic hormone glucagon, which works in opposition to insulin. Glycogenolysis, therefore, elevates blood glucose levels when those concentrations are too low to meet bodily demand. Glycogen stores within a particular muscle cell are available only to fuel chemical processes within that cell and cannot be mobilized to reenter the bloodstream as free glucose.

Excess glucose also can be changed through a series of metabolic processes into fat, or adipose tissue, which consists of three fatty acid molecules bonded chemically to one glycerol molecule. Because of this molecular configuration, fat stores are called triglycerides. Direct consumption and digestion of fats ordinarily will also lead to the formation of triglycerides. Fats, however, are fully interconvertible with carbohydrates.

To be accessible to the muscle cells as an energy source, fats must be broken down into free fatty acids (FFA) through reactions catalyzed by the pancreatic enzyme lipase. A limited quantity of triglycerides is stored within the muscle cells, but these molecules also must be cleaved into FFA to become available for cellular oxidative metabolism.

Proteins are the basic building blocks of human tissue, including muscle tissue. When ingested, animal and plant proteins are broken down by protease enzymes into the amino acid molecules of which they are entirely composed. These amino acids are then reassembled by the body in a multiplicity of configurations determinative of the type and function of tissue formed. Proteins are available as an energy source of last resort and are mobilized only after depletion of both carbohydrate and fat stores. However, when grossly extended exercise or starvation depletes the fat and carbohydrate energy systems, tissue proteins are reduced to amino acids and transferred to the liver, where they are synthesized into glucose through a process called neoglucogenesis. This process appears to be dependent on the action of the hormone cortisol, which is secreted by the adrenal cortex.

Minerals and vitamins are nutrient materials that are absorbed directly through the walls of the small intestine from various food sources. Although they are not directly a source of energy to the body, they are indispensable to the biochemical processes that permit the utilization of carbohydrates, fats, and proteins as energy sources.

ATP: The Body's Fuel

The molecule that appears to be the body's ultimate fuel source in virtually all endergonic reactions, or reactions that consume energy, is adenosine triphosphate (ATP). Adenosine triphosphate consists of two terminal phosphate groups bonded to a nucleotide. The two terminal phosphate bonds in the ATP molecule are energy rich. When one or both of these high-energy terminal bonds is severed, the bonding energy is released and potentially transferred to another molecule, thereby energizing that recipient molecule for participation in further reactions. These exergonic transfer reactions, which release or supply energy, are catalyzed by kinase enzymes. In other words, the energy-rich terminal bonds of ATP provide the primary source of chemical energy that is utilized to fuel endergonic reactions within the body, including those responsible for muscle contraction, nerve impulse conduction, and even energy production itself.

Adenosine triphosphate is produced through a number of chemical pathways, each of which generates a quantity of chemical energy that is captured in the high-energy terminal phosphate bonds of ATP. Most frequently, the synthesis of ATP involves the addition of a terminal phosphate group to a molecule of adenosine diphosphate (ADP). Adenosine triphosphate is not transported from sites of synthesis to sites of activation; rather, it is manufactured within the cells in which it is utilized. Most of the body's cells consequently possess at least one internal mechanism for ATP synthesis.

The principal and most prolific chemical pathway employed by the body's cells to synthesize ATP is called the electron transport system, or oxidative phosphorylation. Oxidative phosphorylation involves the sequential transfer of electrons from one electron acceptor molecule to the next in a series, with oxygen serving as the final electron acceptor. At each step in the electron transport system, the electron passes from a higher energy level to a lower energy level, and that energy differential is partially captured, through enzymatic action, in the high-energy bonding of an additional phosphate group to a molecule of ADP, thereby yielding ATP. After the energy of the electron has been "stepped down" through the electron transport system, the electrons are accepted by molecules of oxygen, which combine with hydrogen ions (also shuttled through the electron transport system) to form water.

Electrons are supplied to the electron transport system for oxidative phosphorylation principally through chemical reactions called dehydrogenations and decarboxylations. These reactions transfer electrons, through enzymatic action, from molecules directly derived from carbohydrates, fats, and proteins to a primary electron acceptor. The most common primary electron acceptors within the body's cells are the pyridine nucleotides—in particular, nicotinamide adenine dinucleotide (NAD) and nicotinamide adenine dinucleotide phosphate (NADP)—and the flavins, especially flavin adenine dinucleotide (FAD). The pyridine nucleotides act as primary acceptors from molecules produced through carbohydrate metabolism, whereas the flavins accept electrons from molecules derived from fat metabolism. These primary electron acceptors then transfer their captured electrons to a series of intermediate electron acceptors, called cytochromes. Finally, the intermediate electron acceptors transfer their captured electrons to oxygen. The electrons that enter the electron transport system by reacting with a primary electron acceptor exist in a higher energy state than the electrons that leave the transport system to combine with oxygen. Much of the energy lost to the electrons is conserved in the synthesis of ATP.

The electron transport system is localized within subcellular organelles called mitochondria, which exist within the cytoplasm of the body's cells. The primary electron acceptors receive most of their electrons from a cycle of dehydrogenation and decarboxylation reactions also localized within the mitochondria. This cyclical series of reactions is called the Kreb's citric acid cycle, or the tricarboxylic acid cycle.

The citric acid cycle begins with molecules of acetyl coenzyme A (acetyl-CoA) derived through the metabolism of either glucose or FFA. Through the complex series of reactions that comprise the citric acid cycle, a total of six electron pairs are transferred to primary electron acceptors for each pair of acetyl-CoA molecules that enter the cycle. The primary electron acceptors then introduce the electrons to the electron transport system, through which a substantial portion of the energy of each electron pair is utilized to synthesis ATP.

The citric acid cycle is not, however, the only system of chemical reactions that transfers electrons to primary acceptors of the electron transport system. The metabolism of a single molecule of glucose into the two molecules of acetyl-CoA that enter the citric acid cycle involves a sequence of two reaction processes, each of which transfers two pairs of electrons to the primary electron acceptor NAD. The metabolism of an FFA molecule into the molecules of acetyl-CoA that enter the citric acid cycle transfers one pair of electrons to the primary electron acceptor FAD. These primary acceptors then shuttle the electrons they have captured to the electron transport system.

The processes of oxidative phosphorylation involved in the electron transport system are the predominant, but not the exclusive, mechanism for ATP production. The initial anaerobic glycolytic processes that metabolize a molecule of glucose into two molecules of pyruvate (which are potentially metabolized into two molecules of acetyl-CoA), generate a net increase of two molecules of ATP. In addition, the metabolism of acetyl-CoA through the processes of the citric acid cycle synthesizes one molecule of ATP for every molecule of acetyl-CoA metabolized. And finally, muscle cells contain a small concentration of creatine phosphate molecules, which, through the severance of their own high-energy phosphate bonds, yield the energy and phosphate groups required to transform ADP into ATP. The anaerobic metabolism of FFA into acetyl-CoA does not directly synthesize ATP.

The Body's Energy Systems

The body's systems of energy production and supply are reflections of these multifaceted metabolic processes. Interestingly, each metabolic system provides an energy source that is relatively specific to a particular energy need. In other words, each distinguishable energy system utilized to supply ATP targets a specific duration and intensity of muscle response.

The energy system that provides the most immediate source of ATP and that consequently provides the primary ATP source for extremely brief but intense exercise is called the alactacid system. It is an anaerobic system (i.e., it produces ATP through processes that do not utilize oxygen), and it involves neither the citric acid cycle nor the electron transport system.

The alactacid anaerobic system utilizes the compound creatine phosphate, which is maintained in limited supply within the muscle cell cytoplasm. The alactacid system generates, through the severance of the phosphate bond in creatine phosphate, the energy necessary to bond that severed phosphate group onto cellular ADP, thereby creating ATP. Although cellular ADP is in abundant supply, the reaction producing ATP from ADP is severely duration limited by the rapid depletion of the cellular supply of creatine phosphate. Any intensive motor response lasting longer than a few seconds (approximately 10 seconds maximum) must rely for production of ATP on some alternative metabolic system.

Once the motor activity is terminated, the alactacid system replenishes its cellular supply of creatine phosphate through the breakdown of ATP into ADP. Experimentation indicates that these creatine phosphate stores are replenished rapidly, such that within 30 seconds of the cessation of work, nearly three fourths of the expended creatine phosphate has been replaced.

The opposing extremity of exercise intensity involves the activity of muscles while the body is at rest. The resting activity of muscles, and even exercise up to moderate levels, can be accommodated by a metabolic process that utilizes fatty substrates as opposed to glucose. In fact, the availability of FFA for cellular metabolism inhibits glucose metabolism at low-intensity exercise. However, as exercise intensity increases, thus causing the ratio of cellular ADP to ATP to increase as energy is consumed in muscle contraction, the inhibition to cellular glycolysis is removed, and carbohydrate metabolism increasingly supplants FFA metabolism as a more efficient energy production system.

The reason for the cellular preference for FFA metabolism in low-intensity exercise and for glucose metabolism in higher-intensity exercise is not fully understood. Fats contain more than twice the accessible energy per gram than do carbohydrates, so the utilization of FFA as a fuel is, in itself, not surprising. Moreover, the energy released through the metabolism of FFA is conserved as ATP almost entirely through the processes of oxidative phosphorylation, suggesting that FFA metabolism is extremely dependent on an availability of oxygen that varies indirectly with exercise intensity. In fact, glucose metabolism produces a slightly higher yield of ATP per quantity of oxygen consumed than does FFA metabolism, supporting the body's increasing preference for glucose metabolism as exercise intensifies.

The first step in the metabolism of fats involves the cleaving of the three fatty acids from the glycerol group to which they are bound during storage. The mobilization of FFA from remote adipose stores is triggered by the hormone norepinephrine, and the FFA then binds with albumin in the blood stream for transport to the muscle cells. The small intracellular, or endogenous, store of triglycerides also must be broken down into FFA for further metabolism.

The FFA is then "activated" through an enzyme-catalyzed reaction that utilizes ATP and is progressively dehydrogenated through a series of reac-

tions that yield a number of molecules of acetyl-CoA, transfe
process, a pair of electrons to the electron acceptor FAD. Oi
of the most common FFA, palmitic acid, will metabolize
molecules of acetyl-CoA. Each molecule of acetyl-CoA then
citric acid cycle, through which one molecule of ATP is synthesized directly, and three pairs of electrons are transferred to a primary electron
acceptor for processing through the electron transport system. The complete metabolism of a "neutral" 18-carbon fatty acid molecule therefore
will yield 147 molecules of ATP. The metabolism of FFA does not appear
rate limited by the availability of FFA substrate. Instead, oxygen availability and enzyme activity appear to be the rate limiting microsystemic
parameters, depending on exercise intensity (see Figure 1).

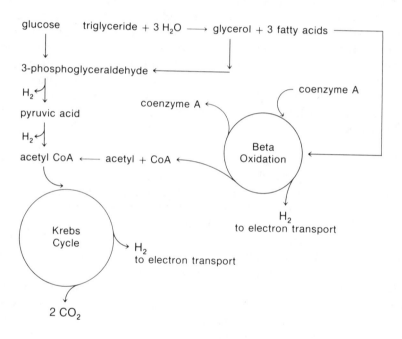

Source	Pathway	ATP Yield per molecule neutral fat
1 Molecule glycerol	Glycolysis + Krebs cycle	22
3 Molecules of 18- carbon fatty acid	Beta oxidation + Krebs cycle	441
		TOTAL 463

Figure 1. The production of ATP through aerobic metabolism of fat. *Note.*
From *Exercise Physiology: Energy, Nutrition, and Human Performance* (p. 97) by
W.D. McArdle, F.I. Katch, and V.L. Katch, 1986, Philadelphia: Lea &
Febiger. Reprinted by permission.

The relationship between glucose metabolism and fat metabolism is governed by a series of intricate chemical feedback loops reflecting exercise intensity. At low-intensity work, fat metabolism spares the use of glucose and can contribute as much as 90% of the muscle fuel needed at rest. With increasing intensity of work, however, the increasing rate of reduction of ATP to ADP and the consequent increase in cellular ADP concentrations feed back progressively to replace metabolism of fatty substrates with glucose metabolism.

Glucose metabolism, or glycolysis, is the principal, though not the exclusive, energy system for fueling exercise of moderate to high intensity. The exogenous form of glucose is stored as glycogen within the liver. Complex hormonal regulatory systems, controlled through the autonomic and the central nervous systems, serve to maintain blood glucose levels within a constant, narrow range. When exercise creates a demand for increased utilization of exogenous glucose, the uptake of glucose from hepatic glycogen is accelerated. Hepatic glycogen is mobilized during exercise by the action of the hormone epinephrine, and hepatic glucose production during exercise can increase to levels as much as 5 times those found during rest. Although exogenous hepatic glucose is not a dominant source of fuel during exercise, it is not insignificant either, as it can contribute as much as one third of the total energy requirement for a given exercise.

Glucose is also stored within the muscle cells as endogenous glycogen. This muscle glycogen is the primary substrate for ATP production during exercise. All strenuous motor tasks that extend beyond the extremely limited capacity of the alactacid system rely primarily upon the reduction of endogenous glucose for the production of ATP.

There are two distinguishable systems that produce ATP through glucose metabolism—anaerobic glycolysis and aerobic glycolysis—and both begin with the same series of chemical reactions.

As with the FFA metabolism, the first step in glycolysis requires the activation of glucose through an enzyme-catalyzed reaction utilizing ATP. Glucose metabolism, however, requires a second activation reaction with ATP to transform fructose-6-phosphate into fructose-1,6-diphosphate. During the further complex series of dehydrogenation reactions that eventually metabolize each glucose molecule into two molecules of pyruvic acid, a total of four molecules of ATP are produced from ADP through the addition of high-energy phosphate bonds. There is, therefore, a net increase of two molecules of ATP during the metabolism of glucose into pyruvic acid. In addition, two pairs of electrons are transferred to the primary electron acceptor NAD during these same chemical processes.

At this point, the reaction can take either of two chemical pathways, depending on the intensity and duration of the exercise involved and, more specifically, on the availability of oxygen. If the exercise intensity is high, the availability of oxygen to the metabolic system will be limited. An oxygen deficiency will manifest in the termination of the electron transport system when oxygen ceases to be available as the ultimate electron acceptor. In a sense, the system simply backs up, preventing the intermediate electron transporters from shuttling the electrons to lower energy levels that already are filled by electrons that can no longer be accepted by oxygen. Under such oxygen-deficient circumstances, the pyruvic acid molecules formed through anaerobic glycolysis become hydrogen acceptors in the place of oxygen, forming lactic acid. Lactic acid accumulates as oxygen-deficient exercise continues, increasingly acidifying the internal cell environment. The processes of glycolysis then slow and eventually cease altogether. Lactic acid can be transported out of the muscle cell into the bloodstream and extracellular spaces, but eventually the purgation process proves inadequate, and the muscle cell reaches a state of terminal acidosis.

At rest, normal muscle fibers have a slightly alkaline pH of 7.08. (A pH of 7 is neutral.) As lactic acid accumulation acidifies the muscle cells, lowering the muscle cells' pH, it interferes with the contractile mechanisms of the muscle fiber and with the functioning of the muscle cells' metabolic processes. Muscle efficiency appears to decrease as a function of the acidity of the muscle cell down to a pH of approximately 6.4, near which point the muscle cell fails. In the process, acidosis of the muscle cell and the surrounding tissues triggers pain receptors located primarily within the connective tissue.

Because anaerobic glycolysis is not rate limited by oxygen availability, the caloric output potential per unit time for this metabolic process is much greater than for the aerobic metabolic systems. Experimentation suggests that anaerobic glycolysis can produce approximately 50% more energy per unit time than can oxidative processes. This, of course, helps to explain why exercise at or near maximum intensity obligates anaerobic metabolism.

After cessation of exercise, a process of recovery begins whereby the acidity of the muscle cells and the bloodstream is neutralized. A small percentage of the lactic acid is converted by the liver back into glucose, but the greatest amount is subjected to a series of aerobic chemical reactions within the muscle cells that convert it to carbon dioxide, water, and energy. The amount of oxygen that is utilized during recovery to oxidize lactic acid and resynthesize glycogen—that is, the amount of oxygen consumed above the volume required for normal resting processes—is commonly referred to as the oxygen debt. The recovery period for the lactacid anaerobic system requires approximately 45 minutes to neutralize the lactic acid accumulations of terminal acidosis. Substantial recovery, including repayment of a large portion of the oxygen debt, occurs far more rapidly. Moreover, the recovery process can be accelerated by the continuation of light exercise. Such a warm-down process seems to speed lactate oxidation and glycogen resynthesis by keeping the circulatory and respiratory systems in a state of elevated activity, thereby facilitating transport of both materials necessary to the regenerative processes and waste products.[1]

The anaerobic lactacid metabolic system, then, is effective only for relatively short and intense episodes of muscle activity. When a highly trained lactacid system is functioning at peak rate, it can persist only for a maximum of approximately 1 to 2 minutes before terminating due to acidosis of the internal muscle environment.

There is, however, a second energy system that is available for exercise of longer duration and lesser intensity. This system, called the aerobic system because it utilizes oxygen, is the primary ATP source for moderate- to high-intensity exercise of any substantial duration.

The aerobic metabolic pathway essentially begins with the two molecules of pyruvic acid produced by the anaerobic metabolism of a single molecule of glucose. The pyruvic acid molecules are subjected sequentially to a decarboxylation reaction that releases carbon dioxide, an intermediate preparatory reaction, and a final dehydrogenation reaction that yields two molecules of acetyl-CoA and two pairs of electrons for acceptance by the primary electron acceptor NAD. The two molecules of acetyl-CoA are then metabolized through the processes of the citric acid cycle, producing four molecules of carbon dioxide, two molecules of ATP, six pairs of electrons that are accepted by NAD, and two pairs of electrons that are accepted by FAD. The complete process of aerobic glycolysis therefore yields for each glucose molecule metabolized a net increase of four molecules of ATP, 10 molecules of NADH, and two molecules of FAD2H. The 10 molecules of NADH release their electrons to the electron transport system, yielding through the processes of oxidative phosphorylation a total of 30 molecules of ATP. Similarly, the two molecules of FAD2H release their electrons to the electron transport system, but at a lower entry level, producing a total of four ATP molecules. In total, therefore, the complete aerobic metabolism of a single molecule of glucose yields 38 molecules of ATP. Approximately 60% of the energy bound in the glucose molecule, however, is lost as heat during the metabolic processes (see Figure 2).

The limiting factor in this energy-rich aerobic metabolic system is the availability of oxygen. As exercise intensity increases beyond a certain threshold, the body's cardiorespiratory capacity cannot supply oxygen to the muscle cells rapidly enough to meet their demands for ATP production. The precise nature of the rate-limiting microsystemic failure in oxygen supply to the muscle cells has not been determined but is suspected to involve either limitations in the heart's capacity to circulate

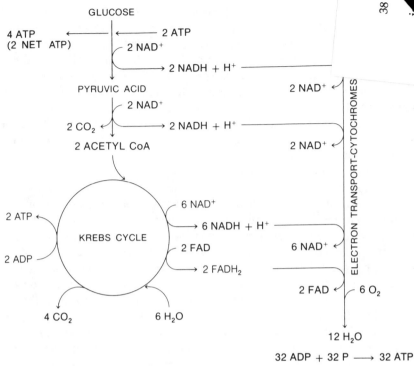

Figure 2. The production of ATP through aerobic metabolism of glucose.
Note. From *Exercise Physiology: Energy, Nutrition, and Human Performance*
(p. 96) by W.D. McArdle, F.I. Katch, and V.L. Katch, 1986, Philadelphia: Lea
& Febiger. Reprinted by permission.

blood-borne oxygen or the overriding increase in oxygen uptake by the
ventilatory muscles as respiration increases beyond a particular threshold.

It appears, to a degree, that individual muscle cells exhibit a preference for either aerobic or anaerobic metabolism. Researchers have identified two principal types of skeletal muscle fiber: slow twitch and fast
twitch. Not surprisingly, the most obvious distinguishing characteristic

the speed with which a particular fiber contracts. Other morphological and physiological differences support this distinction between fiber types in terms of contractile velocity. Slow-twitch muscle fibers—also called red, or type I, fibers—are especially adapted for aerobic metabolism, exhibiting higher internal concentrations of myoglobin and the various oxidative enzymes. Fast-twitch fibers—also called white, or type II, fibers— are better suited for anaerobic metabolism. Physiologists have identified at least two subclasses of fast-twitch fiber, designated type A fast-twitch fiber and type B fast-twitch fiber. Type A fast-twitch fibers appear to be better adapted for aerobic metabolism and less suited for anaerobic metabolism than do type B fast-twitch fibers.

Although each skeletal muscle is a mosaic of all fiber types, the proportion of one type to another is subject to considerable variation from individual to individual. Training does not seem to affect significantly this proportion of one fiber type to another, which appears to be genetically determined. Recent evidence does suggest, however, that endurance training can transform type B fast-twitch fibers into type A fast-twitch fibers, thereby enhancing the fiber's capacity for oxidative metabolism. Moreover, training has been demonstrated to increase dramatically the metabolic efficiency of both slow-twitch and fast-twitch fibers. Improvements in cellular metabolic capacity have been gauged at over 100% for anaerobic fibers and 300% for aerobic fibers. There is recent speculation that the speed of the contractile mechanism within a particular fiber is a function of the size of the activating neuron and that the fiber's orientation in favor of either aerobic or anaerobic metabolism simply reflects its neurally mandated contractile speed.

There are, then, several important performance benchmarks characteristic of the aerobic and the anaerobic metabolic systems. That level of exercise intensity at which the aerobic system is utilized maximally but at which significant lactic acid synthesis and accumulation is not triggered is termed the "anaerobic threshold." It is generally expressed as a measure of the volume of oxygen consumed per unit time.

A second benchmark, termed "maximum oxygen uptake" or $\dot{V}O_2max$, is a measure of the maximum quantity of oxygen that an individual can inhale and assimilate per unit time. Maximum oxygen uptake therefore signifies maximum exercise intensity. Consequently, the anaerobic system is unavoidably implicated during periods of maximum oxygen uptake, causing the production and accumulation of lactic acid and the imminent cessation of such intense exercise.

The production of ATP through the aerobic metabolic system is rate limited by the availability of oxygen supplied by the cardiorespiratory system. Consequently, there are two primary aspects of the aerobic energy system that are targeted with specificity in training. The first aspect is the level of cardiorespiratory activity that permits the aerobic system to operate maximally but beyond which the anaerobic system becomes implicated increasingly as exercise intensifies—that is, the anaerobic threshold. The anaerobic threshold is frequently expressed as a percentage of maximum oxygen uptake. The second aspect involves the speed with which the aerobic system, including cardiorespiratory processes, can be brought to its maximum sustainable level—that is, the speed with which an individual can accelerate the cardiorespiratory system from a state of rest or modest activity to the anaerobic threshold. The predominant limiting factor in the duration of aerobic metabolism appears to be the availability of glucose. In addition, preexercise glucose concentration is believed to have some effect upon the rate of aerobic metabolism.

The anaerobic system operates at a much higher rate than does the aerobic system but is far more limited in duration. Duration of anaerobic metabolism appears limited by acidosis of the muscle cell environment. Training therefore targets the creation and toleration of lactate accumulation in response to exercise at or near maximum cardiorespiratory capacity. The rate-limiting factors in anaerobic metabolism appear to involve preexercise endogenous glycogen concentrations and the efficiency of the enzymatic mechanisms of anaerobic glycolysis. Absolute intensity of exercise lasting longer than 10 seconds presumably is a reflection of rate limitations to the lactacid metabolic process.

The preceding compartmentalization of the energy macrosystem is somewhat artificial; indeed, even the neat distinction between aerobic and anaerobic energy systems is somewhat contrived. Most exercise involves a combination of the three energy subsystems discussed. Exercises characterized as sprints predominantly utilize the alactacid and lactacid anaerobic metabolic systems. Exercises of longer duration increasingly employ the aerobic systems of metabolism. Yet rarely is one metabolic system utilized exclusively.

Training for Endurance

Two basic types of endurance training have evolved, targeting separately the aerobic and the anaerobic metabolic systems. In addition, specific training strategies have been designed to address both the rate-limiting and the duration-limiting aspects of each energy system.

The aerobic metabolic system is most effectively trained through what has come to be called "steady-state" exercise. This genre of endurance training involves either sustained periods of submaximal exercise or intervals of submaximal exercise separated by insufficient rest to permit significant recovery. Proper aerobic training is a quest for the anaerobic threshold. It involves extended periods (e.g., 1 hour) of continuously sustained systemic stress at an intensity approaching the anaerobic threshold.

In short, the aerobic metabolic system must be explored to its limits through practice.

The anaerobic metabolic system is most effectively trained through a system of exercise called *interval training*. Interval training involves relatively short periods of exercise at an intensity above the anaerobic threshold separated by substantial rest periods of varying length. The formula for design of an anaerobic training regimen is somewhat more complex than for aerobic training. Proper anaerobic training in essence is a quest for maximum oxygen uptake. It involves repeated short intervals of maximum- or near-maximum-intensity exercise separated by rest intervals designed to permit a specific degree of recovery. Maximum-intensity exercise of 1 to 2 minutes is sufficient to accelerate the cardiorespiratory system to maximum oxygen uptake, producing incipient muscle failure. The length of rest intervals and the number of exercise intervals are varied along with the length of exercise intervals in order to produce a specific training effect. Inadequate rest intervals, or an excessive length or quantity of exercise intervals, will transform anaerobic training into aerobic training. Ultimately, the anaerobic system must be explored to its limits through practice.

An episode of maximum- or near-maximum-intensity exercise must commence with anaerobic energy production and supply. During the period in which the cardiorespiratory system accelerates toward maximum oxygen uptake, the burden of energy supply falls upon the lactacid—and for a few seconds only, the alactacid—anaerobic systems. For intensive exercise lasting longer than approximately 1 to 2 minutes, anaerobic metabolism must be replaced increasingly by the aerobic metabolic system. Exercise longer in duration than 1 to 2 minutes, therefore, will be submaximal in intensity and increasingly will involve the utilization of aerobic metabolism. The shorter the rest interval and the greater the number of exercise intervals during a single training session, the less able will be the anaerobic system to sustain maximum intensity exercise and the sooner the intensity will fall to a level at which it can be sustained aerobically.

There are, of course, a multiplicity of subtle variations on these two broad genres of endurance training. Design of training regimens is far from a well-settled science. To be sure, physiologists attach numbers to such training parameters as maximum oxygen uptake and the anaerobic threshold. Yet for any particular training session, such benchmarks of the energy systems are definable and accessible only subjectively. The athlete must tune into the subtle combination of bodily experiences that attend the exercise with sufficient specificity and intensity to explore each macrosystem and microsystem functionally implicated to its limits in failure.

Strength and Power: The Contractile Mechanism

Muscle response is governed not only by limitations in endurance but also by limitations with respect to strength and power. The aerobic and the alactacid and lactacid anaerobic metabolic systems are the mechanisms by which muscle contractions are energized and are therefore indispensable and integral to the strength and power of a muscular contraction. Training specific to the energy systems, however, targets muscle endurance rather than strength or power.

The muscle is the basic organ of movement. The skeletal muscles, through contractions within a skeletal structure of joints and bones, are responsible for nearly all voluntary bodily movements. The basic mechanism of muscular contraction is partially understood and is believed to be common to all muscle, including skeletal, smooth, and cardiac tissue types.

Each muscle fiber consists of a cell membrane, or sarcolemma, enclosing several nuclei and a mass of myofibrils and other organelles bathed in cytoplasm. Each myofibril consists of a longitudinal chain of patterned segments called sarcomeres. The sarcomere is the integral unit of contraction. Each sarcomere consists of myofilaments of two proteins: actin and myosin. The organization of the actin and the myosin filaments is regular. Each sarcomere possesses two bundles of actin filaments, separated from one another in the center of the sarcomere and originating from the membranelike boundaries of the sarcomere with adjacent sarcomeres. The opposing ends of a single bundle of myosin filaments are interdigitated into the facing but separated bundles of actin filaments, thereby bridging the longitudinal gap between the actin filament bundles.

The myosin filaments are thicker than the actin filaments and possess minute molecular projections that form crossbridges during the contractile process to reactive sites on the smooth, thinner actin filaments. Each myosin filament, where it is interdigitated with actin filaments, is surrounded by six, hexagonally oriented actin filaments. The myosin filaments are aligned to form regular crossbridges to all six surrounding actin filaments. The resultant pattern of interdigitation causes each actin filament to receive crossbridges from three, triangularly oriented myosin filaments (see Figure 3).

Contraction of the sarcomere involves a telescoping of the actin filament bundles toward one another along the myosin filament bridge. The myosin filament bundle remains stationary, and the facing ends of the actin filament bundles effectively slide toward one another along the increasingly interdigitated myosin filaments. Neither the myosin filaments nor the actin filaments shorten in length. The telescoping contraction of the actin filaments toward one another along the longitudinal myosin

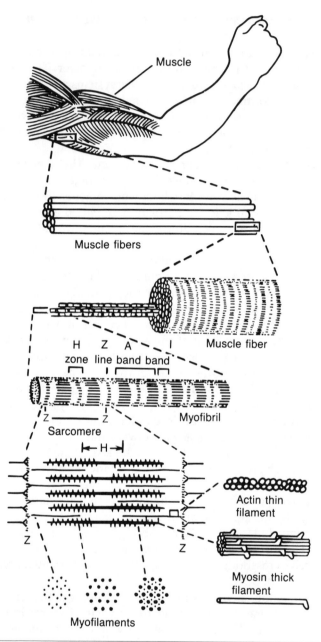

Figure 3.   A schematic dissection of skeletal muscle. *Note.* From *Human Physiology* (2nd ed., p. 195) by A.J. Vander, J.H. Sherman, and D.S. Luciano, 1973, New York: McGraw-Hill. Reprinted by permission.

filament bridge, however, shortens each sarcomere (and therefore the muscle fiber) by as much as one third.

The precise chemistry of the contractile mechanism has not been determined, but a relatively detailed model of that process has been hypothesized. Each myosin filament appears to possess a head and a tail. The tails, called light meromyosin, bind together to constitute the main filament length. The heads, called heavy meromyosin, project out from the filament length in a highly regular pattern. The actin filaments, on the other hand, are two elongated protein molecules combined in a double helical formation with reactive sights oriented in the same regular geometrical configuration as the heads projecting from the myosin filaments. When the fiber is relaxed, the actin filament reactive sites contain negatively ionized ADP and the proteins troponin and tropomyosin. These chemical agents, through their bonds with the actin filament, inhibit molecular crossbridging between the actin and the myosin filaments (see Figure 4).

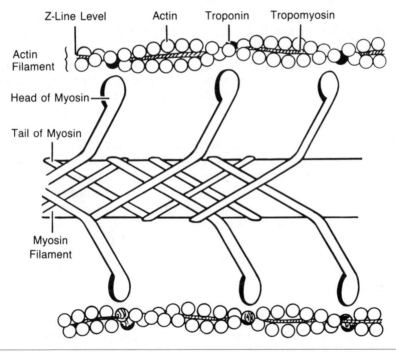

Figure 4. The molecular structure and relationship of the actin and myosin filaments. *Note.* From *Training for Sport and Activity* (3rd ed., p. 9) by J.H. Wilmore and D.L. Costill, 1988, Dubuque, IA: Wm. C. Brown. Reprinted by permission.

The base of the heavy meromyosin projection is negatively charged and contains the enzyme ATPase, whereas the tip of the projection contains negatively ionized ATP. In the resting state, the negative charge at the base of the projection repels the negatively charged tip of the projection, causing the projection to extend out at an oblique angle from the myosin filament. The neuronal excitation of a muscle fiber causes the introduction of positively charged calcium ions into the sarcomere from the sarcoplasmic reticulum. Troponin, through a reaction involving tropomyosin, binds the calcium ions, thereby releasing the inhibition on crossbridging between the actin and the myosin filaments. The resultant crossbridge reaction between the extended tip of the meromyosin projection and the reactive site on the actin filament depolarizes the tip of the myosin filament projection, causing an electrostatic contraction of that projection. Because the myosin filament projections extend at an oblique angle to the filaments, the contraction of the projection pulls the actin filament longitudinally with respect to the myosin filament. This process of contraction brings the ATP localized in the tip of the myosin filament projection into contact with the enzyme ATPase localized at the base of that projection. The action of ATPase on ATP produces a chemical reaction that reduces ATP to ADP, releasing energy that cleaves the molecular crossbridge to the actin filament. The ADP molecule is then replaced by a negatively ionized ATP molecule supplied from cellular energy systems, and the heavy meromyosin projection is again electrostatically extended at the same oblique angle. This cycle repeats, at a frequency as high as 100 times per second, so long as calcium and ATP are available, and the actin filaments are, in a sense, ratcheted along the myosin filaments.

Figure 5 is a highly schematic diagram of the hypothesized cross-bridge mechanism. A cross-bridge extension of the myosin filament attaches to a receptive site on the actin filament (top), and then undergoes a configurational transformation that causes the actin filament to slide incrementally along the myosin filament (middle), resulting in a new orientation of the actin and myosin filaments that triggers a chemical change that cleaves the cross-bridge (bottom). Asynchronous cross-bridge reactions sustain the contractile process during a particular gross episode of contraction.

The purgation of calcium ions from the sarcomeres back into their bound state in the sarcoplasmic reticulum triggers relaxation of the muscle fiber and is believed to involve a system of active transport. Therefore, ATP is presumed to be involved as an energy source not only in the actual contractile process but also in the molecular pumping mechanisms that purge calcium from the contractile unit, allowing the fiber to relax.

The tension generated within a single sarcomere through this contractile process is understood to vary, depending on the number of crossbridges implicated at any one time. Consequently, the greater the degree

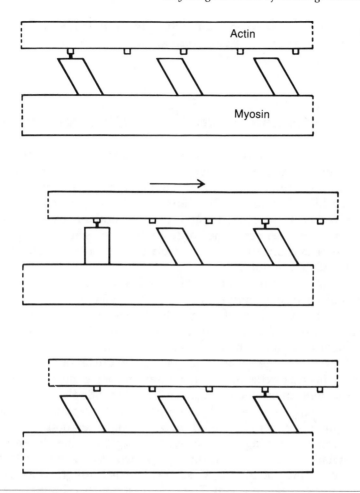

Figure 5. A schematic diagram of hypothesized cross-bridge mechanism. *Note.* From "Molecular Basis of Contraction in Cross-Striated Muscles and Relevance to Motile Mechanisms in Other Cells" (p. 42) by H.E. Huxley in *Muscle and Nonmuscle Motility, Volume I,* edited by A. Stracher, 1983, New York, Academic Press. Adapted by permission.

of interdigitation of actin and myosin filaments within a sarcomere, the greater the tension generated within that sarcomere through crossbridge cycling. Any overlapping of the actin filaments at the center of the sarcomere through extreme contraction, however, appears to obstruct crossbridging to some degree, resulting in a decrease in contractile tension.

Contractions are classified in the following categories: isometric, in which there is no active shortening of the muscle fiber during contraction; isotonic, or concentric, in which the contraction actively shortens the muscle fiber; and eccentric, in which the muscle fiber lengthens as it attempts to contract against an overpowering force. All involve the same basic mechanism of contraction.

Neural Mechanisms Involved in the Contractile Process

Each muscle fiber is coupled to a motor neuron through a mechanism called the motor end plate. In anatomical areas involving fine muscle control, such as the fingers, eyes, and tongue, there are few muscle fibers connected to each neuron; but in areas involving gross motor control, such as the back and the upper legs, one motor neuron can excite hundreds of muscle fibers. The entire excitatory mechanism, consisting of the motor neuron, the motor end plate, and the innervated muscle fibers, is called a motor unit.[2]

The excitatory stimulus comes from the neuron to the muscle fiber in the form of a neuronal impulse. The neuromuscular junction is not, however, a direct connection of neuron to muscle cell. Just as successive neurons are separated from one another by synaptic spaces or gaps, so too the neuromuscular junction is actually a synaptic gap. Neuronal impulses must bridge the synaptic gap in order to excite contraction within the muscle fiber. The chemical agent for transmission of neuronal impulses across the neuromuscular synapse has been identified as acetylcholine, or ACh, which is synthesized in the presynaptic region of the motor neuron, and appears to be stored there in conglomerations or vesicles. A nerve impulse arriving at the presynaptic region excites the entry into the presynaptic terminal of calcium ions, which react with proteins within the presynaptic membrane to open channels through which ACh is perfused into the synaptic gap. The ACh then diffuses across the synaptic gap to reach receptor sites located on the postsynaptic muscle cell membrane. The action of ACh on the muscle cell membrane results in the depolarization of that membrane sufficiently to propagate an impulse or action potential along the muscle fiber membrane in the same way conduction occurs along the neuronal axon. The localized depolarization of the muscle fiber to its action threshold consequently results in the propagation of an action potential in both directions along the muscle fiber's length. The ACh within the synaptic cleft is then hydrolized by enzyme action and recycled to the presynaptic site for resynthesis and storage as ACh. Meanwhile, the action potential generated along the muscle cell membrane causes a release of calcium ions into the fiber cytoplasm that in turn binds troponin, thereby releasing the inhibition on crossbridging between the actin and the myosin filaments. The rapidity of the conduction of the action potential in both directions along the muscle fiber enables relatively synchronous contraction throughout the entire fiber length.

There does not appear to be variation in the intensity (as distinct from the duration) of contraction within a single muscle fiber. Either it contracts with full intensity or it does not contract at all. All of the muscle fibers within a single motor unit, however, do not necessarily contract and relax in unison. The frequency of neuronal impulses reaching the neuromuscular junction determines the amount of neurotransmitter that reaches the individual muscle fibers. If that frequency is low, it is possible that some of the muscle fibers within a motor unit will reach their action threshold, and others will not. When the frequency of neuronal impulse to the motor unit is high, all the fibers within the motor unit will be driven to their action thresholds.

A single action potential within the muscle cell will cause only a single contractile burst, or "twitch," followed by relaxation. However, if the stream of action potentials transmitted across the neuromuscular gap occurs so rapidly that insufficient time is allowed for the muscle to relax, the contraction will be sustained, or tetanized. The intensity of contraction by any single motor unit is governed by the rapidity of neuromuscular transmissions to the muscle fibers up to a maximum frequency beyond which transmission is precluded by the nerve cell's refractory, or recovery, period. Once a motor unit is flooding the synaptic gap with ACh through peak frequency impulse propagation, additional contractile strength can be achieved only by the recruitment of additional motor units.

Virtually all skeletal muscles are continuously maintained in a state of slight contraction, called tonus, produced by continuous low-level stimulation by impulses from the motor neurons. Tonus is believed to involve alternating stimulation of the many motor units within a muscle, such that a low-level muscle contraction is sustained without burdening any single group of fibers. Tonus, in addition to providing general postural support to the skeleton, maintains the muscles in a state of readiness from which they are able to contract with greater speed, coordination, and strength.

In addition to excitatory neuronal impulses, which cause muscle fibers to contract, impulses propagated by certain nerves inhibit muscle contraction. Inhibition apparently occurs within the neuromuscular gap and involves the presynaptic release of a neurotransmitter that either directly or indirectly increases the polarization of the postsynaptic muscle cell membrane, effectively raising the action threshold of that membrane.[3]

Neural control, therefore, is of cardinal importance to the processes of muscular contraction. By the recruitment of specific motor units for contraction and by signaling the rate of contraction, the neuronal coding becomes fundamentally determinative as to muscle strength, power, and endurance.

Training for Strength and Power

Just as sophisticated training systems have been developed to enhance the endurance of muscle response, so too have highly refined training systems evolved to enhance muscular strength and power. These training systems involve the exercise of a specific, relatively isolated muscle group through a predetermined range of contraction against a predetermined resistance.

Strength, which is a measure of the force that is exerted by a single muscle contraction, is best trained by high-resistance, low-repetition exercise regimens. Pure strength training, targeting a specific muscle group and contractile motion, would consist of a single maximum contraction. With rare exceptions, this is not a realistic way to train. Yet low-repetition, high-resistance exercise has been determined to be the most effective training scenario for sheer strength improvement.

Power training addresses both the strength and the velocity of the muscle contraction. Power increases achieved through training have proven to be relatively rate specific. Low-velocity strength increases, for example, are not particularly transferable to high-velocity strength applications. There is somewhat greater transferability of high-velocity strength gains to lower-velocity strength applications, but approximate rate specificity still obtains for power training. Simply put, power training at a given contractile velocity tends to increase power primarily for that general contractile velocity. Consequently, the efficacy of power training is maximum when the contractile speed in strength training is kept approximately equal to the contractile speed ultimately desired in performance.

Because contractile speed necessarily decreases as resistance increases, power training requires a balance between the level of resistance and the velocity of contraction. Pure strength training, irrespective of contractile velocity, requires training against maximum resistance. This requires a determination of the maximum strength capability of the muscle group to be trained. Pure speed training, irrespective of contractile strength, requires training at maximum contractile speed against minimum resistance. This requires a determination of the maximum speed capability of the muscle group to be trained, together with a determination of the level of resistance that begins to slow the muscle contraction. Pure speed training frequently will entail techniques of artificially minimizing resistance, such as running downhill. Power training, however, requires a determination of the contractile power capability of the muscle group to be trained, a measurement combining strength and velocity. Power training that emphasizes strength enhancement therefore requires maintenance of the minimum acceptable contractile speed during exercise against the maximum possible resistance. Power training that emphasizes speed enhancement, on the other hand, requires maintenance of the minimum acceptable resistance against exercise performed at maximum contractile velocity. Consequently, power training generally involves lower-resistance, higher-repetition exercise at higher contractile velocity than does pure strength training.

Only the specific muscles that are stressed through training reflect a significant training benefit. In fact, strength and power training are specific to the individual muscle fibers recruited to achieve the particular range and intensity of contraction involved in the training exercise. Training therefore is specific as to the range, strength, and power of contraction.

Training specific to the performance parameters of strength, power, and endurance also are, to a degree, specific to either fast-twitch or slow-twitch muscle fiber types. Pure strength training, consisting of high-resistance, low-repetition exercise, increases the size of (or "hypertrophies") the slow-twitch fibers and increases their contractile strength without triggering physiological adaptations that increase slow-twitch fiber endurance. In fact, slow-twitch fiber hypertrophy appears to have a detrimental effect on both slow-twitch fiber endurance and fast-twitch fiber power due to the increase in muscle bulk. Power training increasingly implicates the fast-twitch fibers as contractile speed increases. Fast-twitch fibers are trained for strength by high-resistance, low-repetition exercise at high contractile velocity. Strength increases in fast-twitch fibers usually involve some concomitant fiber hypertrophy, but principally of the fast-twitch fibers. Fast-twitch fibers are trained for speed by low-resistance, medium- to high-repetition exercise at maximum contractile velocity. Slow-twitch fiber endurance is most effectively trained by low- to moderate-resistance, high-repetition exercise specifically targeting the rate and duration limitations of the aerobic metabolic system. Fast-twitch fiber endurance is most effectively enhanced through moderate-resistance, moderate-repetition training targeting the rate and duration limitations of the anaerobic metabolic systems. Neither aerobic nor anaerobic endurance training appreciably hypertrophies or strengthens the muscles.

The distinction between fast- and slow-twitch muscle fibers, however, cannot be taken too far. As explained above, physiologists have identified two subclasses of fast-twitch fibers, and there are indications that even finer divisions of fiber type may be appropriate. Eventually, individual muscle fibers may be revealed to possess contractile speeds and oxidative propensities that range all the way from slow twitch to fast twitch and are not substantially limited to the two extremes. Currently, however, the division between slow-twitch, fast-twitch type A, and fast-twitch type B fibers appears to be an acceptable approximation of discernible fiber types.

The Principle of Right Practice

Take infinite pains to make something that looks effortless.
Michelangelo

There are three general laws of physical training that can be extracted from the practices that have been developed to train the energy, contractile, and neuronal macrosystems. The practices from which these general principles are derived have evolved through subjective experience compounded over generations of athletic training, and their efficacy has been verified not only in the crucible of competition but recently in the scientific laboratory.

The first and fundamental postulate is the principle of Right Practice. The second and third postulates are actually refinements of this first principle of Right Practice. They are the rule of specificity of practice and the rule of intensity of practice.

The principle of Right Practice is universal and absolute. Quite simply, the principle of Right Practice recognizes that progress in any discipline necessarily involves Right Practice of that discipline.

The Rule of Specificity of Practice

The rule of specificity of practice takes the principle of Right Practice one step further. It holds that the degree of progress attained through the practice of a discipline is directly related to the degree of specificity with which the practice reflects the discipline.

This rule is exemplified in the training of the body's energy microsystems. Steady-state training, which stresses the aerobic system almost exclusively, produces cellular adaptations that improve the functioning of the aerobic system. There appears to be only incidental training benefits to the anaerobic system through strict aerobic training. Interval training, which places maximum stress on the anaerobic system, produces physiological changes that facilitate and enhance the anaerobic system. Because anaerobic training necessarily involves maximum cardiorespiratory stress and because the aerobic system is responsible for replenishing the oxygen debt accumulated through a period of anaerobic exercise, anaerobic training indirectly benefits the aerobic metabolic system. However, this training effect is limited and difficult to manage. It does not violate the rule of specificity; rather, it is a reflection of the fact that anaerobic exercise unavoidably implicates aerobic mechanisms.

The rule of specificity is even more apparent in the training methods targeting strength and power. In the first place, training benefits are extremely specific as to the muscle fiber exercised. Training through contraction of a specific motor unit does not train neighboring units. Training the left arm does not train the right. Muscle training also is specific as to both velocity of contraction and contractile range. So, for example, strength gains achieved through isometric exercise, in which the range and velocity of contraction are absolutely limited by an equal, opposite resistance, are not fully transferable to contractions of the same fibers at lesser or greater contractile lengths. Strength- and power-training regimens properly attempt to isolate specific muscle groups and to exercise those muscle groups through a predetermined range of contraction at a predetermined speed. The contractile range and speed selected for training are designed to approximate the range and speed desired in the ultimate performance. The greater the specificity of the training, the greater will be the training effect. The training benefit, of course, will be limited substantially to the specific muscle movements involved in the training.

The Rule of Intensity of Practice

The second refinement of the principle of Right Practice is the rule of intensity of practice. Simply stated, the rule of intensity of practice holds that the degree of progress attainable through the practice of a discipline is directly related to the intensity of the practice.

This rule also is readily understood in relation to the training of the body's energy systems. Subjective experience, confirmed by scientific investigation, has established that the beneficial effect of system-specific training on either the aerobic or the anaerobic metabolic system is directly related to the intensity with which the respective training modes are approached.

There are two dimensions of intensity for both aerobic and anaerobic training: rate and duration. In aerobic or steady-state training, intensity is a function of the aerobic metabolic rate that is sustained for the duration of exercise. Maximum-intensity aerobic training involves maintenance of exercise intensity at a level approaching the anaerobic threshold until glucose stores are depleted. In anaerobic or interval training, intensity is a function of the anaerobic metabolic rate achieved and sustained over repeated intervals separated by rest. Maximum-intensity anaerobic training involves the achievement and maintenance of maximum oxygen uptake for each successive exercise interval to the limits of terminal muscle cell acidosis.

The rule of intensity of practice is nowhere better reflected than in the area of strength and power training. Subjective experience has taught, and scientific investigation has verified, that training potentially stimulates numerous molecular adaptations in the muscle cells, resulting in an increase in the strength and power of the fiber's contraction. The rapidity and degree to which such adaptations occur correlates directly with the intensity of training.

Rarely do athletes achieve maximum intensity in training or even in competition. There is no question, however, that the degree of intensity of practice is directly related to the training benefit achieved. Right Practice of course must accommodate the recovery and rebuilding needs accompanying high-intensity training, and rest therefore is an essential element in the design of a training regimen.[4] With the proper combination of specific and intense practice and adequate rest, a training regimen will produce numerous physiological adaptations to the energy systems and contractile mechanisms.

Physiological Adaptations in Response to Right Practice

According to the principle of Right Practice, a desired performance standard is most effectively pursued through a system of training that targets both the specificity and the intensity of that performance standard. The proper application of the rules of specificity and intensity of practice gives rise to pervasive and dramatic physiological adaptations that enhance physical performance.

In response to Right Practice targeting muscular endurance, the most critical and identifiable physiological changes occur within those microsystemic mechanisms that are limiting to each energy system's production of ATP. The rate-limiting aspect of the aerobic system, which obligates anaerobic metabolism for high-intensity work, involves the availability of oxygen to the aerobic metabolic pathway. This appears to be a function of ventilatory capacity, and physiologists have confirmed that cardiorespiratory mechanisms for oxygen uptake are substantially enhanced through aerobic training. Among the more pronounced and easily measurable gross physiological changes accompanying aerobic training are the following: increased cardiac output; increased pulmonary ventilation; increased red blood cell count, as well as increased hemoglobin content within the red blood cells; increased blood volume and distribution; and increased vascularization of the muscle fibers. Numerous more subtle changes at cellular and subcellular levels also have been documented to accompany aerobic training, including the following: increased intracellular glycogen storage and myoglobin concentrations, especially within the slow-twitch fibers; proliferation of mitochondria within the slow-twitch fibers; transformation of type B fast-twitch fibers into type A fast-twitch fibers, thereby enhancing their oxidative capacity; facilitation of the hormonal and enzymatic processes involved in the mobilization of hepatic glycogen and exogenous FFA; and enhancement of enzyme activity related to oxidative metabolism, especially of the various mitochondrial enzymes involved in both the citric acid cycle and the electron transport system. More than 50 specific intracellular adaptations have been identified to correlate with aerobic training.

The limitation on duration of aerobic exercise appears related primarily to glucose availability. Aerobic metabolism within a highly trained muscle will continue until glucose stores are depleted. Thereafter, exercise can be sustained on metabolism of fatty substrates—and aerobic training facilitates the systems involved in FFA mobilization and metabolism—but only at a reduced intensity. Not surprisingly, therefore, the mechanisms involved in the storage and supply of glucose to muscle fibers are extremely susceptible to enhancement through training. Not only does aerobic training substantially enhance the activity of the hormonal and enzymatic agents that mobilize and transport glucose to the muscle cells from hepatic glycogen stores, but endogenous glycogen concentrations are increased dramatically as well. Moreover, steady-state training that emphasizes the duration limitations of the aerobic metabolic system enhances the activity of the hormone cortisol, thereby facilitating gluconeogenesis, a process through which proteins are converted to glucose. A common example of a training strategy designed to increase glucose supply is known as "carbohydrate loading." This process, whereby supercompensation in the resynthesis of muscle glycogen is triggered through dietary manipulations accompanying exercise that depletes glycogen stores, can more than double the muscle fiber's preexercise concentration of endogenous glycogen.

The principal limitation on the anaerobic metabolic system is one of duration and appears to be related primarily to the acidification of the muscle cell environment. Physiologists have demonstrated that the cellular processes that oppose acidosis in the muscle cell are enhanced substantially through proper anaerobic training. In addition, lactic acid toleration is improved through such training. The rate-limiting factors in anaerobic metabolism are not well understood, but analysis has substantiated a wide range of intracellular changes resulting from anaerobic training. Many of these adaptations parallel the transformations attendant on aerobic training but are localized within fast-twitch rather than slow-twitch fibers. For example, the following cellular adaptations within fast-twitch fibers have been correlated with anaerobic training: enhancement of the activity of the hormones and enzymes that are rate limiting to the anaerobic glycolytic processes that transform glucose into pyruvic acid; increased concentrations of endogenous glycogen, ATP, and creatine phosphate; and facilitation of the hormonal and enzymatic processes for mobilization of hepatic glycogen. And on a macrosystemic level, cardiorespiratory functions, which are stressed maximally through anaerobic training, exhibit dramatic improvement in response to such training. These physiological adaptations that facilitate anaerobic metabolism do not seem to have any deleterious effect on cellular aerobic metabolism.

The physiological adaptations that accompany strength and power training appear to be equally as pervasive and dramatic. Probably the most obvious microsystemic transformation in response to pure strength

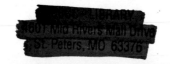

training involves the hypertrophy of the slow twitch muscle fibers, causing a potentially immense increase in overall muscle size. Although recent evidence suggests that there is some longitudinal splitting of muscle fibers, the actual number of fibers does not appear to change significantly in response to strength or power training, even when fiber hypertrophy is extreme. Within the muscle fiber, a number of physiological adaptations have been correlated with strength and power training, including the following: an increase in the number of myosin and actin filaments; an increase in the ratio of myosin filaments to actin filaments, with possible increases in the thickness of the myosin filaments; enhancement of the enzymatic processes involved in crossbridge cycling; and facilitation of the active transport process that purges calcium ions from the sarcomere. Moreover, to the degree that a particular power-training regimen emphasizes contractile speed over pure strength, that training scheme increasingly will implicate aspects of endurance training, especially those related to the anaerobic metabolic processes. Consequently, power training also will tend to increase endogenous ATP, creatine phosphate, and glycogen concentrations and will facilitate the anaerobic glycolytic system.

The adaptive potential of the cardiorespiratory system and of the many chemical processes transpiring on the molecular level within the muscle cells provide a firm physiological foundation for physical training designed to enhance the performance parameters of strength, power, and endurance. However, the muscle fiber's profound dependency upon neural excitation suggests that the nervous system is vitally implicated in control of the energy and contractile macrosystems that are more immediately determinative of those performance parameters. As explained previously, there are two principal aspects to neural control of the energy and contractile mechanisms. First, the selective recruitment of motor units is governed by neural mechanisms. Second, the contractile force generated within each recruited motor unit is neurally controlled. The characteristic neural response to a maximally strenuous motor task will involve the following scenario: an initial selective recruitment of motor units; an elevation of neuronal impulse frequency to these recruited motor units in order to maximize the contractile response of the constituent muscle fibers; and a progressive recruitment of additional motor units to increase the net contractile force up to maximum performance capability. Neural recruitment of motor units can be either haphazard and inefficient or highly purposeful and efficient. Proper training will increase the efficiency of neural recruitment. Because recruitment patterns will vary tremendously depending on the performance parameter emphasized, the facilitation of neural recruitment is specific to the training system utilized. For example, although anaerobic power training emphasizing a high contractile velocity will facilitate neural recruitment of type B fast-twitch fibers, aerobic strength training will predominantly facilitate neural recruitment

of slow-twitch fibers. The selection and progressive recruitment of motor units therefore can be patterned with specificity through training. In addition, it appears that the attainment of maximum neuronal impulse frequency to recruited motor units is facilitated, again with specificity, by physical training.

As already indicated, there is also a neural system of inhibition at work within each motor unit. Each muscle fiber appears to interface at its synaptic junction with both an excitatory and inhibitory nerve. Although the specific function of this inhibitory neural system is not fully understood, it is clear that neuronal disinhibition, as well as excitation, can be patterned with specificity through training.

All of these neural mechanisms—impulse frequency to selected motor units, selective recruitment of motor units, and disinhibition of motor units—are therefore subject to the rule of specificity of practice and the rule of intensity of practice. Ultimately, the two rules operate in symbiotic harmony, and the enhancement of the efficient selection and exploitation of motor units becomes a function of the intensity of the specific practice.

Right Practice: In Pursuit of Failure

The increased frequency of neuronal impulses to mobilized motor units and the progressive recruitment of additional motor units are responses to the failure of those fibers already mobilized for contraction to meet the strength, power, or endurance demands of exercise intensity. Increases in fiber recruitment and mobilization, therefore, are a consequence of an intensity of training that exceeds the performance capacity of a prior level of fiber mobilization. The enhanced activity of the energy and contractile systems also is a direct consequence of training that drives those systems to their physiological performance limits.

The performance limitations of the various energy systems—whether of rate or duration—are most effectively extended through training in which system-specific energy demands exceed those limits. Similarly, the performance limitations that inhere in the physiology of the contractile mechanisms appear to be extended through training that places strength and power demands on the fiber in excess of those performance limits. limits.

The performance parameters of strength, power, and endurance, therefore, all are most effectively trained through exercise programs that take the performance-limiting physiological microsystem to failure. Whether the training regimen is designed to increase strength through low-repetition, high-resistance exercise or to increase power or endurance through some configuration of lesser resistance and higher repetitions, the performance-limiting physiological system must be identified with specificity and trained to failure. There is no other meaningful gauge available for assuring that training intensity is adequate to stimulate the many physiological adaptations that increase performance capability. In other words, the many specific enhancements to the energy and contractile macrosystems are presumed to be a result of the proper exercise of each particular system. Training methods attempt to target the likely point of failure within each physiological system and to exercise around that point. Progress comes in the precise discipline that is practiced and to a degree that directly reflects the intensity of practice. Points of failure in all instances define the limits of systemic function. Right Practice must seek to extend those limits through the pursuit of failure.

Failure, conceived in this way, is a point of physiological incapacity within the energy, contractile, or peripheral neural macrosystems. It involves, then, the cessation of systemic function due to a breakdown in some electrochemical process, or microsystem, integral to the failing macrosystem. The closer to the failure of physiological incapacity a specific functional system is extended, the greater the training benefit to that system.

Failures involving the cessation of systemic function due to physiological incapacity are the essence of Right Practice. Each such moment of failure becomes a success in its passing. Objective performance criteria employed to determine an order of finish in a training exercise or competition and to define objective standards of excellence potentially distract the practice from a proper focus on the pursuit of systemic failure. Yet without question, the rewards for competitive success are extremely potent seductions to practice ardently and correctly. Consequently, a focus of awareness on the rewards for competitive success within a discipline of body can be utilized to direct and inspire Right Practice. However, awareness must not be occupied with such rewards during actual, formal periods of practice. In other words, there is an operant distinction between periods of formal practice, oriented toward systemic failure, and periods of nonpractice, frequently oriented toward some objective success. Outside the formal practice, physical training involves the pursuit of success. Within the formal practice, physical training involves the pursuit of failure.

Notes

[1]Replenishment of the body's glycogen stores, however, ordinarily requires a far longer time period than lactate purgation. Depending upon diet and exercise levels during the recovery period, replacement of substantially depleted glycogen stores can take one to several days.

[2]See chapter 5 for a detailed analysis of the neural mechanisms involved in motor response and of neurophysiology generally.

[3]The smooth muscles of the body, which comprise the walls of the hollow internal organs and blood vessels, are most frequently under inhibitory control.

[4]These writings do not attempt to design specific training programs, and the critical subject of rest and recovery needs is one of the paramount design considerations not addressed.

4

A Physiological Model of
Mind: The Theory

*The meaning of the message will not be found in the chemistry of
the ink.*

R.W. Sperry

To this point, the concept of coordination has been defined on two levels.
First, the willpower of the mind was conceived as a force field arising
out of the mind's focus in an image of purpose, and that force field was
understood to modulate the forces of determinism to ''co''-''ordinate''
a particular state of body. Although the states of body analyzed in
chapters 2 and 3 were principally those states associated with complex
motor performance, states of body also were understood to include the
physiological states of the brain. The first definition of coordination therefore involved the coordination of states of body by states of mind.

This bold concept of coordination, then, was hypothesized to be an
essential feature of Right Practice. As explained in chapter 1, it is the concept of purpose that distinguishes practice from simple experience.
Chapter 2 expanded on this proposition by theorizing that the focus of
the mind as an image of purpose potentially is reflected in the specificity
and intensity of practice. The image of purpose, in other words, is understood to radiate a force field, focused alternatively as volition and attention, that has the capacity to modulate the forces of determinism that
otherwise would dictate experience. By formulating an image of purpose

and by encoding that image into physiological processes such as neuronal conduction and muscular contraction, the mind becomes the author of practice. The mind, in this respect, is potentially autonomous and is distinguishable from the strictly deterministic physiological processes of the brain, the body, and the phenomenal universe.

The second level of definition of the concept of coordination, set forth in chapter 2, concerned the integration and sequencing of various states of body. The mind was not directly and immediately implicated in this conception of coordination. Instead, coordination was analyzed as but one of four discernible parameters of performance, all of which were revealed to be proximately determined by the multiple peripheral physiological microsystems integral to the subject motor performance. The performance parameter of coordination, however, was left relatively neglected, as the chapter's focus targeted the more easily measurable and quantifiable performance parameters of strength, power, and endurance. Nonetheless, coordination emerged as fundamentally determinative of the three subsidiary performance parameters subjected to scrutiny. And under analysis, the neuronal macrosystem was revealed to be the physiological agency of such coordination. Through its multiple constituent microsystems, the neuronal macrosystem was revealed to recruit, mobilize, integrate, and sequence the myriad of functional microsystems integral to complex motor performances.

This chapter explores in greater depth the distinction between these two conceptions of coordination. The ultimate question is whether the neuronal macrosystem is potentially "coordinated" by the mind, as contemplated in the Theory of Right Practice, or whether it is "self-coordinating" and strictly subject to the laws of mechanistic determinism. It is obvious, of course, that the subjective manifestations of mind are closely associated with the physiological processes of the brain. Is there, however, any meaningful distinction between the mind and the brain? The threshold question, in other words, is whether the mind can be explained solely in terms of the physiological processes of the neuronal macrosystem.

The relationship of the incorporeal mind to the corporeal body has been the subject of philosophical inquiry and empirical investigation for virtually all of recorded history. There are two fundamentally antithetical explanations of the relationship of the mind to the body, and both have persisted through history to the present day. These two explanations are commonly termed *monism* and *dualism*.

Monism, which also is referred to as identity theory and reductionism, views the mind as essentially indistinguishable from the physiological processes of the brain. The subjective states of awareness described by such terms as *purpose, volition, attention,* and *will* all are understood to be mere passive epiphenomena associated with the physiological processes transpiring within the central nervous system. The mind, therefore, is postulated to have no causal effect on the physiological processes of the brain, although it is understood to arise entirely as an incorporeal effect of those corporeal processes.

Dualism, on the other hand, views the mind and the brain as fundamentally distinguishable. Some modern dualists view the mind as not entirely incorporeal but as consisting of such subtle organizations of matter and energy as to be undetectable and unmeasurable given present instrumentation. Others who subscribe to the dualist faith simply perceive the mind to be an aspect of some incorporeal spirit or soul that acts upon the corporeal universe through mechanisms that are unknown and possibly unknowable, except, perhaps, subjectively.

During the last several decades, scientific empiricism has made tremendous progress in understanding the physiological processes of the central nervous system. There is strong evidence now that the subjective states of awareness—including volition, attention, and will—correspond precisely to particular physiological processes. The monists have embraced this empirical evidence to support their hypothesis that subjective awareness is nothing more than a passive epiphenomenon attendant upon the physiological processes of the brain. And indeed, the evidence is persuasive. By modifying states of the brain—as, for example, through neurosurgery or the administration of pharmacological agents—researchers unquestionably have produced certain correlative and predictable modifications of states of mind. The degree to which states of subjective awareness are alterable by manipulations of brain architecture and chemistry seems to compel the conclusion that states of mind are determined by states of brain. The dualists, of course, respond with compelling subjective "proof" of the preeminence of mind and its potential to "determine" states of brain and body. But subjective proofs are proofs of nothing within the framework of Western empiricism. Subjective experience, after all, is hypothesized by the monists to be simply an impotent epiphenomenon associated with the organic machinery of the brain.

At the outset of this inquiry into the nature of the mind, then, it appears that the path of Western empiricism is predestined, by virtue of its own first principles, to confirm the reductionist paradigm that relegates the mind to the status of an inconsequential effect of the brain. And, of course, there is no meaningful notion of practice within such a conceptual paradigm. By now, this should come as no surprise. Already, the Western empirical path to Right Practice has been predicted to be a dead end. Yet just beyond that dead end lies the realm of pure mind, and the border zone between the objective corporeal universe and the subjective universe of the mind is posited as the field in which Right Practice transpires. To reach that field of practice, then, the Western path to a Physiological Model of Mind must be followed to its end.[1]

The Neuronal Macrosystem

Not so long ago only vague hobbits inhabited the land of neuro-mythology.

Karl Pribram

The path to a Physiological Model of Mind begins, not surprisingly, with the neuron. The physiological microsystems integral to neuronal conduction, both within the neuron and across the synapses that connect individual neurons into a neuronal network, combine to convey information throughout the body. They also are presumed to constitute the functional substrate of the brain. These physiological processes that give rise to neuronal conduction involve complex electrochemical reactions most clearly discernible on the cellular and molecular levels. There are two general categories of microsystems, each comprised of linked chains of electrochemical reactions, that are involved in the conduction of a neuronal impulse.

First, there are processes that transpire within the nerve cell that cause an "action potential" to propagate through that nerve cell and especially along the nerve cell's primary conductive tract, called the axon. The propagation of the action potential is dependent on the flow of electrically charged ions through the nerve cell membrane. Molecular "gates" within the membrane control the ionic current, but the gates themselves also are responsive to variations in electrical charge. The neuronal impulse is propagated within the nerve cell in discrete bursts that reflect the sequential opening and closing of the molecular gates progressively along the cell membrane. The opening and closing of these molecular gates is triggered by the electrical charge that precedes the progression of the action potential. In other words, the action potential associated with the ionic current passing through the molecular gates within the nerve cell membrane produces a leading "wave" of electrical current that triggers the successive membrane-gating microsystems, thereby causing the progressive propagation of action potentials along the membrane. This leading electrical wave, however, cannot be sustained without being constantly regenerated by the processes of the action potential it triggers. The microsystemic processes that produce the action potential exhibit a brief "refractory" period, in which they are inoperative, following each episode of propagation.

The second fundamental category of microsystems of neuronal conduction involves conduction across the synapses between individual neurons. The classical synapse involves an actual space, or synaptic gap, between nerve cells. When the action potential reaches the presynaptic terminal, it must be conveyed across the synaptic gap in order to initiate an action potential in the postsynaptic nerve cell. Synaptic transmission occurs primarily through the operation of neurotransmitters that convey the neuronal impulse across the synaptic gap. The arrival of an action potential in the presynaptic terminal causes molecular gates to open in the presynaptic nerve cell membrane, through which the neurotransmitter is perfused into the synaptic gap. The neurotransmitter then diffuses across the synaptic gap and reacts with receptor sites on the postsynaptic nerve cell membrane. Nerve impulse conduction is achieved when the reaction at the postsynaptic membrane initiates an action potential in the postsynaptic nerve cell.

There are, then, two fundamental parameters to the physiological processes of neuronal conduction. First, neuronal conduction is coded through the frequency of impulse conduction. Frequency refers to the number of impulses, or action potentials, generated at a single locus during a given period of time. Second, neuronal conduction is coded in terms of the spatial conformation of the conductive pathway. This second parameter for neuronal coding is governed primarily by the processes involved in synaptic transmission. The microsystemic linkages between nerve cells, in other words, join discrete nerve cells into a unified network of neuronal conduction.

These two parameters for coding neuronal impulses—frequency and conformation—have the capacity to encode a virtually unlimited quantity of information. The sophistication of this binary coding system is reflected, for example, in the coordination of complex motor activity. As discussed in chapters 2 and 3, the spatial conformation of neuronal conduction recruits specific muscle fibers for contraction, and the frequency of neuronal conduction determines the intensity of the contraction. Here, then, within the information codes of the neuronal system, are embodied the two dimensions to Right Practice: specificity, reflected in the neuronal recruitment of specific muscle fibers for contraction; and intensity, reflected in the frequency of neuronal transmission governing the intensity of the muscle contraction. From complex schemes of neuronal conduction to muscle fibers throughout the body, the most astoundingly sophisticated motor performances are coordinated.

This binary code reflected in the performance parameter of coordination is determined, however, by a prior level of coordination, and the physiological processes integral to this prior level are presumed to transpire principally within the brain. The brain is a highly complex organization of neurons, glial cells, and other tissues, fluids, and spaces. It is, in essence, an electrochemical milieu that virtually defies morphological or physiological explication. Despite the enormous efforts of generations of researchers, scientific understanding of the brain remains quite limited. There is, however, near universal agreement regarding certain basic assumptions about the ways in which the brain functions. Among these accepted tenets of neuroscience is the presumption that the binary code of neuronal and synaptic transmission is the primary modality of brain function. The microsystems involved in propagation of the action potential within the nerve axon and those microsystems implicated in the transmission of neuronal impulses across the nerve synapses are presumed to constitute the two principal processes that give rise to functional states of the brain, including states of mind.

Perhaps the most significant of the common suppositions regarding brain function is the understanding that virtually all of the brain's processing functions, whether sensoric or motoric in nature, implicate multiple brain centers. Although various areas of the brain have been revealed to be functionally specific, any significant processing function requires the integration of a multiplicity of such localized functional areas. Dr. Wilder Penfield, a pioneer of modern neurosurgery, characterized the brain's integrative processing modality as "centrencephalic integration." Although Penfield distinguished between the pathways of centrencephalic processing associated with automatic and autonomic functions and those associated with conscious functions, he concluded that virtually all brain functions involve substantial centrencephalic integration.

Penfield was, of course, entering the realm of speculation in proposing distinct centrencephalic processing mechanisms for automatic and conscious functions. Yet such a distinction seems patently plausible, and numerous other scientists and philosophers have entered that same inviting realm. After all, it is only reasonable that the profound qualitative distinction between subjective awareness and automatic functions should be a reflection of distinguishable physiological processes.

The available information relating to the mechanisms of higher brain function (limited though it might be), when combined with the more extensive morphological evidence relating to brain architecture, suggests the existence of specific physiological processes that may be integral to consciousness—an approximate Physiological Model of Mind. This model is premised on evidence that conscious awareness corresponds to a dynamic, sustained transcortical electrochemical process. Awareness, in other words, can be hypothesized to involve specific physiological elaborations of Penfield's centrencephalic integration.

The Hyperneuronal Arc of Awareness

> *Mind comes into action and goes out of action with the highest brain mechanism, it is true. But the mind has energy. The form of that energy is different from that of neuronal potentials that travel the axon pathways. There I must leave it.*
>
> Wilder Penfield

In his popular book *The Brain*, Dr. Richard Restak (1979) briefly describes a model of consciousness developed by Dr. E. Roy John, director of the Brain Research Group at New York University, in which the electrochemical processes of centrencephalic integration are conceptualized as "hyperneurons." The processes of consciousness, including the subjective sense of awareness, are modeled by John as epiphenomena accompanying electrical energy processes spanning a network of neurons, glial cells, and other brain tissue and spaces. It is these patterned electrochemical interactions propagating through the brain medium that constitute hyperneurons, and John hypothesizes that "the content of subjective experience is the momentary contour of the hyperneuron." The existence of the hyperneuron has not been confirmed experimentally, and even John recognizes that his correlation of subjective experience and the hyperneuron is extremely speculative. Yet John takes this speculation even further to suggest that "subjective experience may actually be a property of a certain level of organization in matter" (Restak, 1979).

In such general form, John's hypothesis of the hyperneuron, provocative as it seems, takes the Physiological Model of Mind little further than the imagery of Penfield's centrencephalic integration or even Sir Charles Sherrington's poetic conception of the brain as an "enchanted loom." There exists, however, an evidenciary basis for a substantial, informed elaboration of these admittedly speculative conceptions of the physiology of awareness.

To begin with, then, the Physiological Model of Mind assumes that the hyperneurons associated with conscious awareness are transcortical electrochemical phenomena. Yet experimental evidence suggests that much of the processing involved in complex sensory and motor functions, including those functions characterized as voluntary or conscious, takes place in highly localized processing centers. Visual and somatic processing, for example, appears to involve periodic columnar subdivisions of the cortex measuring approximately 1 millimeter in diameter and 2 millimeters in depth. One such column of neocortical cells will perform a highly specific function, and must be integrated with numerous other neocortical cell ensembles similarly localized as to function, frequently across wide expanses of neocortical gray matter, in order to effectuate coordinated sensory perception or motor response. It is the centrencephalic integration of multiple localized functions that constitutes the hyperneuron in the Physiological Model of Mind.

The hyperneuron, perceived in this way, becomes a gestalt phenomenon in which the transcortical centrencephalic processing that integrates discrete patterns of neuronal conduction creates a unified physical system with properties that transcend those of the constituent parts. Most commonly, such transcortical centrencephalic processing is regarded as sequential in nature. And, for automatic and autonomic functions, sequential processing through multiple stages of localized cell groupings is plausible. However, sequential processing seems inadequate to explain the gestalt of conscious awareness that attends certain transcortical manifestations of centrencephalic integration. Instead, hyperneurons associated with conscious awareness are best understood to involve a simultaneity of processing, such that the unified physical system that constitutes the hyperneuron exists at once in time and in space. The transcortical conduction pathways associated with awareness therefore do not reflect localized electrochemical activity (such as an action potential or burst of action potentials) projected through a patterned sequence of local processing centers to terminate in some unknown brain region that triggers awareness. Awareness is more reasonably presumed to be the ''emergent'' subjective property attendant on the unified, simultaneous manifestation of a particular sustained transcortical hyperneuronal arc: the *hyperneuronal arc of awareness*. The hyperneuronal arc of awareness is conceived in this context as an integrated, unitary phenomenon in time and space, in which localized processing functions traversed by the hyperneuronal arc are simultaneously alive in electrochemical resonance.

The hyperneuronal arc therefore is suggested to be a unified, simultaneous, sustained episode of transcortical neuronal conduction. The state of subjective awareness attendant on the hyperneuronal arc has an ''emergent'' quality, meaning that the ''whole'' of subjective awareness exceeds the sum of the physiological ''parts.'' In other words, the hyperneuronal arc simultaneously implicates a spectrum of physiological microsystems within widespread regions of the brain, and the result of this simultaneous linkage is not the mere quantitative summation of functional microsystems but is the qualitative leap to subjective awareness.

This is not to suggest, however, that such hyperneuronal arcs do not arise through some sort of sequential processing. Instead, it demands that localized processing functions be sustained rather than transient and merely sequential so that the hyperneuronal arc might manifest at once in its entirety. Assuming that a hyperneuronal arc arises sequentially, then—even if from multiple diffuse origins along convergent pathways—that arc is consummated when electrochemical conduction along the pathways described by the arc is sustained at least long enough for the initial or leading impulses to traverse the full arc before impulse propagation along that arc is terminated. Hyperneuronal arcs, of course, may be sustained beyond this minimum period necessitated by the presumption of simultaneous processing. Yet in the Physiological Model of Mind, each episode of consciousness requires at a minimum the momentary existence of a unified hyperneuronal arc.

With the conceptualization of a transcortical hyperneuronal arc as the suggested physical manifestation of awareness, questions immediately arise as to the spatial conformation of such arcs within the brain. Several general observations can be made relative to the spatial configuration of hyperneuronal arcs of awareness. First, the processes of neuronal conduction appear to be unidirectional. That is, conduction appears to be limited to a single direction for any particular axon or synapse. Second, electrochemical conduction within the neocortical gray matter apparently is organized in terms of small, localized functional areas that are not necessarily integrated horizontally throughout a particular gyrus, or convolution. Conduction integrating two or more convolutions appears most frequently to require the use of the various association tracts lying beneath the sheet of cortical gray matter. Although a generalized electrical conduction across the neocortical sheet is not impossible, it seems far more likely that integration of multiple gyri implicates the deeper short and long association tracts within the cortical white matter. The hyperneuronal arc, consequently, may emerge as a process of unidirectional electrochemical conduction in which the arc's spatial configuration reflects the integration between gyri through deep tracts of cortical white matter and the integration of local functional areas within each implicated gyrus through conduction processes insinuated within the cortical gray matter.

This, of course, is not to suggest that hyperneuronal arcs of awareness arise as singular, unidirectional, sequential processes of conduction sustained over time. Experimental evidence suggests, in fact, that the hypothesized hyperneuronal arc must involve multiple convergent systems of neuronal conduction originating in diffuse locations both internal and external to the brain. Neuronal impulses generated at multiple peripheral sensory portals, involving both exteroceptor and proprioceptor organs, converge on the brain, where they are integrated with impulses generated through "spontaneous" discharge from various centers within the brain to produce the cohesive, unitary gestalt of conscious awareness.

Both conscious and automatic brain mechanisms are understood to utilize systems of centrencephalic integration to orchestrate complex motor and sensory responses. The electrochemical hyperneurons associated with conscious awareness should be distinguishable physiologically from those processes of neuronal conduction that give rise to automatic and autonomic (i.e., nonconscious) behavioral responses. Indeed, the majority of human motor response and sensory reception occurs without attendant subjective awareness. Even the most complex motor skills, once learned, can be performed (usually better) with little or no subjective volition. Similarly, highly sophisticated sensory screening routinely is performed without the attendance of subjective attention. Yet there remains a profound qualitative distinction between brain functions attended by subjective awareness and brain functions that transpire without conscious awareness.

The most likely basis for distinguishing between conscious and automatic centrencephalic integration is the extent to which the particular conduction pathway involves neocortical and subcortical gray matter and especially the frontal and temporal lobes of the cortex. The subjective sensations of volition and attention appear to correlate with detectable transcortical electrical potentials. Moreover, the frontal and temporal lobes have been demonstrated to be the cortical regions critically involved in functions related to the formation of purpose or intent and to the storage and retrieval of memory, respectively. The automatic and autonomic processes, on the other hand, appear to involve a far more limited expanse of neocortex, implicating primarily only the appropriate sensory and motor regions of the cortex, vertically integrated with multiple lower-brain centers. Therefore, although complex motor response and sensory reception not attended by subjective awareness does involve the functional integration of relatively widespread regions of the brain, these neuronal processes appear to involve far less extensive cortical regions than do those implicated in subjective awareness. Moreover, the neuronal processing underlying motor response and sensory reception that does not involve subjective awareness appears to be sequential in nature rather than simultaneous as in conscious response and perception.

Binary Coding in the Hyperneuronal Arc

> *The mathematician G. H. Hardy is supposed to have said a mathematician is someone who not only does not know what he is talking about but also does not care. Those who discuss in depth subjects such as the physiology of the mind probably care, but I cannot see how they could ever know.*
>
> David H. Hubel

The hyperneuronal arc of awareness, although conceived as a discrete physiological phenomenon, is but an episodic embodiment of the microsystems implicated in neuronal conduction. The microsystems integral to the propagation of the action potential within the nerve cell combine with the junctional microsystems integral to synaptic transmission to create a transcortical electrochemical arc. This hyperneuronal arc therefore exhibits the same binary code encountered in the peripheral neuronal macrosystem. One aspect of this binary code is the external conformation of the hyperneuronal arc, which is a reflection of the microsystemic linkages between neurons, whereas the second aspect is the internal frequency of the hyperneuron, which is a reflection of the microsystemic propagation of neuronal impulses. Although it is relatively obvious that the frequency codings have virtually unlimited variability, it is also true that configurational codings are quite fluid. In other words, the neural network is not "hard wired."

The microsystemic linkages between neurons within the central and peripheral nervous systems—and especially those concentrations of synaptic and ephaptic junctions contained in the various gray matter centers within the brain—are understood to operate not as switchboards or digital processing stations for impulse propagation but as analogue processing centers. The nature of the processing function is dependent on the electrochemical milieu that is generated as the medium for synaptic and ephaptic conductance. These microsystemic linkages are understood to be extremely susceptible to modification. In fact, the junctional mediums are sculpted in substantial part by the very impulses that they process. These impulses are understood to originate either in the receptor fields of the numerous sensoria or in "spontaneous" discharges from neural centers within the brain.

A particular microsystemic linkage between neurons is created by the episodic perfusion of neurotransmitter into the synaptic gap from the convergent presynaptic terminals. The temporal and spatial summation of the excitatory and inhibitory transmitters comingled within the synaptic cleft determines the nature of the junction and its processing effect. Changes of variable durability in the gating mechanisms of the presynaptic and postsynaptic terminals in response to the passage of neuronal impulse currents (and perhaps also changes in the activity of the enzymes that compose and decompose the neurotransmitters) provide the basis for the molecular changes in the microsystemic linkages that give rise to long- and short-term memory. Some researchers have even speculated that the junctional microsystems potentially include chemical reactions comparable to the embryogenetic process of induction, whereby a splitting of the glial surround occurs to permit the growth of entirely new neuronal junctions.

In other words, the processes by which memory is encoded within the brain are hypothesized to involve principally the modification of the microsystemic linkages joining the neurons within the brain into a particular transcortical conductive network. Although it is certainly probable that the physiological adaptations associated with the encoding of memory also produce organic modifications affecting the conduction of the action potential within the neuron, the more dramatic and discernible molecular changes associated with memory occur at the synapses. The physiological adaptations associated with memory appear to facilitate a specific pattern of neuronal conduction, and this adaptive facilitation appears to result from prior episodes of neuronal conduction in that same pattern. The evidence suggests, in fact, that conceptual memories are encoded *only* as a result of episodes of neuronal conduction attended by subjective awareness. Neuronal conduction not accompanied by subjective awareness will not precipitate the kinds of physiological adaptations within the microsystemic linkages that are believed to encode conceptual memory.

The Physiological Model of Mind is premised on the centrencephalic integration of discrete neuronal microsystems that are organized and integrated through modifiable microsystemic linkages. The hyperneuronal arc of awareness is therefore understood to embody a binary functional modality. The frequency of propagation of action potentials within the constituent neuronal microsystems determines one parameter of the binary code of a particular hyperneuronal arc. The conformation of the hyperneuronal arc, as mandated by the junctional microsystems within that arc, determines the second parameter of the binary code. Both parameters are variable.

Dr. Karl Pribram, a prominent neurosurgeon and neuropsychologist, has formulated a theory of brain function that emphasizes this binary code of neuronal transmission. Specifically, Pribram delineates "a two-process coding mechanism of brain function consisting of a state and operations on that state." The "state" is the momentary conformation of the neural network, involving both the "fast potential" neural macrostructure and the "slow potential" junctional microstructure. The "operations on the state" are the frequency codings of the neuronal impulses that traverse and describe that conformation within the moment (Pribram, 1981, pp. 95-96).

French neurobiologist Jean-Pierre Changeux, in his recent book *Neuronal Man: The Biology of Mind* develops a "biological theory of mental objects" that also emphasizes the binary nature of information coding and processing within the brain:

> *The mental object is identified as the physical state created by correlated, transient activity, both electrical and chemical, in a large population or "assembly" of neurons in several specific cortical areas. This assembly, which can be described mathematically by a neuronal graph, is discrete, closed, and autonomous, but not homogeneous. It is made up of neurons possessing different singularities . . ., laid down in the course of embryonic and postnatal development. . . . The earmark of the mental object is thus initially determined by the mosaic (or graph) of neuronal singularities and by a state of activity in terms of the number and frequency of impulses flowing in the circuits they form* (Changeux, 1985, pp. 137-138).

There are, then, two principal parameters hypothesized to define a particular hyperneuronal arc: the spatial conformation of the arc within the three dimensions of brain space, and the frequency of impulse conduction within that arc. The spatial configuration of a given hyperneuronal arc is conceived in most instances to be convergent, irregular, and delimited. Theoretically, therefore, each such arc possesses a definite episodic existence in time and space, determined by the microsystemic linkages between neurons. The boundaries in space of a hyperneuronal arc constitute the external focus to that arc. The second critical parameter to the hyperneuronal arc is the frequency of neuronal impulse conduction. Because the amplitudes of action potentials appear to be invariant, neuronal impulses are presumed to be coded entirely by frequency. The sustained frequency of impulse conduction along a hyperneuronal pathway determines the intensity of that arc and constitutes its internal focus.

A hyperneuronal arc can be generated either by afferent sensory impulses originating outside of the brain or by faculties lying within the brain. In either case, the hyperneuronal arc originates in diffuse, discrete neuronal phenomena that coalesce in associative patterns and relationships, ultimately converging into a unified, compound whole. The coalescence from diffuse processes to a single, unified process involves the focusing of the hyperneuronal arc. That focusing occurs simultaneously on both the internal and external levels and culminates in a hyperneuronal arc of a particular external spatial conformation and internal frequency.

The Physiology of Conceptual Awareness

Indeed, no scientist, by virtue of his science, has the right to pass judgment on the faiths by which men live and die. We can only set out the data about the brain, and present the physiological hypotheses that are relevant to what the mind does.

Wilder Penfield

The hyperneuronal arc, therefore, is posited as the physiological basis of mind. The subjective sensation of awareness, whether arising as attention or as volition, is modeled as an epiphenomenon attendant on each physical manifestation of hyperneuronal arc. It follows that variations in the nature of awareness arise as reflections of variations in the nature of the hyperneuronal arc. Consequently, an analysis of the patterns of correspondence between states of awareness and physiological brain states is extremely revealing.

The point of departure for this investigation involves the understanding that awareness arises in consciousness only and always as conceptualization. Conceptualization, in other words, is the *sine qua non* of conscious awareness. Conceptualization, of course, consists of the formation of concepts. Concepts, in this broad sense, include all manifestations of abstract thought. Without concepts, the mind is empty and cannot rationally be considered to exist. The Physiological Model of Mind hypothesizes that the internal and the external focuses to the hyperneuronal arc are entirely determinative of the conceptualization that will arise in conscious awareness. Not surprisingly, then, the binary physiological processes underlying the hyperneuronal arc are understood to be reflected in the conceptualizations to which they give rise.

Hyperneuronal arcs arise through a process of convergence of diffuse electrochemical activity into a delimited, unified process. Although the process of coalescence can be conceived frequently to begin in the peripheral proprioceptor and exteroceptor organs of the various sensoria, it will suffice to analyze that process as it transpires within the brain. Each neuronal impulse that enters the brain through afferent tracts, and each impulse generated within the brain itself, presumably will be processed through a particular pathway of conduction. At that point of initial presence within the brain, whether originating there or entering on afferent fibers, the neuronal impulse is an isolated, discrete event. Differentiation, or dissociation, therefore, is maximum at that point of origin of neuronal activity within the brain. From this maximum level of dissociation, all processes of centrencephalic integration proceed. Integration occurs through the association of the previously diffuse neuronal impulses into a coherent, unified process of conduction. Integration and association culminate in the formation of those transcortical hyperneuronal arcs attended by conceptual awareness. Each hyperneuronal arc therefore is an association of neural activity defined entirely by its internal and external focuses. Those same focuses, however, simultaneously differentiate that arc from all others.

Conceptualization, like the hyperneuronal arc of awareness, also arises through simultaneous differentiation and association. Conceptualization involves the fragmentation of the experiential universe into discrete things and events, called concepts. Every concept is an aggregate of other concepts. A conceptual "object" refers to this aggregate, whereas a conceptual "process" refers to the interactions between conceptual objects. Conceptual objects and processes are associated with and differentiated from one another in terms of conceptual "properties." Properties are the conceptual terms that define a conceptual object or process as a distinguishable, approximately autonomous state of matter and energy in space and time. Each conceptual object or process, therefore, is defined, associated, and distinguished in terms of the conceptual properties that impose on a configuration of matter and energy a conceptual framework of space and time. The conceptual framework of space and time both differentiates and associates at once, as conceptual objects and processes arise together in conceptual awareness. As differentiation approaches absolute fragmentation of the phenomenal universe, however, the fragments of conceptual differentiation become increasingly uniform and less sharply measurable, rendering the criteria for distinguishing one from another increasingly ineffectual until they fail altogether. Similarly, however, as relationships between fragments approach absolute association, the units of conceptual association become increasingly less distinguishable from one another until there is no longer any discernible "thing" to associate. Just as the hyperneuronal arc is conceived as possessing a definite, coherent configuration in time and space, so too do all concepts possess a delimited conformation in time and space. A concept can no more be diffuse and unbounded that can the hyperneuronal arc to which it is presumed to owe its existence.

Concepts, therefore, are differentiated and associated simultaneously in terms of properties, thereby defining and delimiting an object or process in time and space. In the Physiological Model of Mind, the conceptual properties that simultaneously define and distinguish conceptual objects and processes can be understood to arise in awareness as a function of the binary coding of the hyperneuronal arc. The spatial conformation of the hyperneuronal arc—that is, its external focus—determines the spatial delimitation of the corresponding concept. The frequency of the hyperneuronal arc—that is, its internal focus—determines the temporal delimitation of the corresponding concept. Just as each hyperneuronal arc arises always as a synthesis of external and internal focuses, so too do concepts arise always as a synthesis of spatial and temporal boundaries. The degree of focus to conceptual awareness is a function of the degree of resolution of the conceptual parameters of time and space, which are themselves determined by the internal and external focuses to the arc of awareness.

The spatial parameter to conceptualization implies the manifestation of concepts as corporeal objects or things. Inherent in the definition of spatial properties is the presumption that some "thing"—some object or product—can be delimited within the three dimensions of space. The concept of "matter" arises to describe such spatially definite objects within conceptualization. The temporal parameter to conceptualization implies the manifestation of concepts as processes reflecting energy or force. Temporal properties define the processes of change that inevitably and incessantly affect matter. The concept of "energy" arises to describe such processes of transformation within conceptualization.

It bears reiteration that the temporal and spatial properties of awareness arise always in the unified synthesis of a particular concept. The dimension of time is meaningless except in the context of the dimensions of space, and the dimensions of space are meaningless except in the context of the dimension of time. Similarly, the concepts of matter and energy arise always in indivisible unity. The Physiological Model of Mind, which postulates the hyperneuronal arc as the physical embodiment of awareness, suggests the process according to which such intimately paired concepts as space and time, and matter and energy, can be understood to arise.

In an ultimate sense, the spatial dimensions of any particular concept are cognizable only in terms of the temporal dimension, and the temporal dimension is cognizable only in terms of the spatial dimensions. Cognition of either the spatial or the temporal dimensions must occur in terms of properties that are susceptible to measurement. Such properties, therefore, are expressed in terms of standards of measurement corresponding to some reference object external to the property to be measured. The properties constituting the spatial dimensions, consequently, are measurable and therefore cognizable only by reference to standards of measurement embodied within the temporal dimension. Similarly, the properties constituting the temporal dimension are measurable and cognizable only by reference to standards of measurement embodied within the spatial dimensions. Ultimately, the spatial and temporal dimensions are defined and delimited only through a fundamentally relativistic process of reciprocal definition.

In the Physiological Model of Mind, this reciprocity of measurement and cognition inherent in conceptualization is understood to be a direct reflection of the relationship between the internal focus and the external focus of the hyperneuronal arc of awareness. When the internal focus to the arc remains constant as the external focus fluctuates, the invariant frequency of that internal focus becomes a standard of measurement in reference to which the variant spatial conformation of the external focus can be determined. Alternatively, when the external focus to the arc of awareness remains constant as the internal focus varies, the invariant spatial configuration of the external focus becomes a standard of measurement in reference to which the variant frequency of the internal focus can be determined. Conceptualization ultimately arises through such a process of reciprocal cognition of the complementary dimensions of space and time, reflecting the underlying functional reciprocity of the external and internal focuses to the hyperneuronal arc of awareness.

The Physiological Model of Mind, extrapolated to this extent, suggests that all concepts are fundamentally relative. Concepts, in other words, have no absolute meaning but instead are defined entirely in relationship to other complementary concepts. Such an absolute relativity of conceptualization is understood to be a direct reflection of the complementary relationship between the external and the internal focuses to the hyperneuronal arc of awareness. Consequently, concepts arise only in complementary pairs, of which space and time and their correlates, matter and energy, are archetypical.

The absolute relativity of conceptualization also reflects the binary nature of the microsystemic neural processes integral to the hyperneuronal arc of awareness. According to the present theory, the hyperneuronal arc is an electrical process involving the molecular conformation of atoms and the flow of ionic currents across nerve cell membranes. The electromagnetic force underlying all electrical phenomena involves the interaction of positive and negative electrical charges. The mutual "attraction" of positive and negative electrical charges and the mutual "repulsion" of like charges are the basic forces governing the electrochemical interactions between atomic elements. Similarly, the ionic currents that conspire to propagate neuronal impulses are positive and negative divergencies from a dynamic equilibrium of electrical charge. The point of dynamic equilibrium is the midpoint or balance point between the equal opposing divergencies of positive and negative charges. Positive and negative electrical charges, consequently, are understood to be fundamental complementary physical properties that are defined entirely through their reciprocal relationship.

In the Physiological Model of Mind, the binary processes of the brain also are understood to give rise to two complementary modes of subjective awareness: attention and volition. Although the distinction between attention and volition occasionally may seem clouded, it most often is clear and unambiguous. At any rate, conceptualization arises always in awareness oriented to some degree either as attention or volition. Traditionally, such a dichotomy of orientation is hypothesized to correspond to the distinction between states of conceptual awareness attendant on processes of sensory perception (i.e., attention) and states of conceptual awareness accompanying motor response (i.e., volition). Sensory perception and motor response, however, are not mutually exclusive processes. Motor response is integral to sensory perception (as, e.g., in directing and focusing the eye), and sensory perception is indispensable to motor response (as, e.g., in the biasing of muscle spindles). Consequently, the Physiological Model of Mind distinguishes between attention and volition in terms of whether the state of subjective awareness is understood to consummate or initiate an approximately autonomous body of sensory-motor processes. Attention involves those receptive sensory-motor processes by which patterns external to mind are imported as hyperneuronal arcs of conceptual awareness. Volition involves those projective sensory-motor processes by which hyperneuronal arcs of conceptual awareness are exported to a universe external to mind. Attention and volition, then, are the complementary and reciprocal functional modes of the mind.

The Great Truth of Adaequatio

> But although all our knowledge begins with experience, it does not follow that it arises from experience. For it is quite possible that even our empirical experience is a compound of that which we receive through impressions, and of that which our own faculty of knowledge (excited only by sensuous impressions), supplies from itself, a supplement which we do not distinguish from that raw material, until long practice has roused our attention and rendered us capable of separating one from the other.
>
> Immanuel Kant

In the suggested Physiological Model of Mind, cognition is understood to be a direct reflection of the physiological processes that give rise to transcortical hyperneuronal arcs of awareness. From this perspective, it follows that the brain creates a mental conception of the phenomenal universe in its own image. The physical processes of cognition, in other words, entirely determine the conceptual awareness of reality. Yet only insofar as these internal physiological processes of the brain are congruent with the external physical processes of the phenomenal universe can the mind be conceived to cognize an external reality.

It is, of course, quite reasonable to assume that the physiological processes of the brain do not differ from the physical processes external to the brain. After all, the process of evolution is widely accepted as an external process that created the internal processes of the brain in its own image. Such reasoning, however, is unconvincing, for the conception of evolution as a model for the origin of the processes of mind is itself a product of those processes of mind. Not surprisingly, therefore, the model of evolution displays the same internal relativity and complementarity as all other manifestations of conceptual awareness. This relativity is most obvious in the law of natural selection, which is hypothesized to govern the otherwise random processes of evolution. The law of natural selection is adequately and succinctly encapsulated in the phrase "survival of the fittest." Fitness, however, is defined entirely and retrospectively in terms of survivability: A species survives because it is fit, yet it is fit because it survives. A model of evolution premised on such a patently relative law cannot be employed to suggest that there exists some definite and absolute reality external to conceptual awareness.

Nevertheless, a conceptual model of an external phenomenal universe, as well as a Physiological Model of Mind, arise within subjective awareness. The relationship between the internal realm of conceptual awareness and the external realm of a physical reality is the quintessential philosophical issue. The hyperneuronal arc of awareness has been hypothesized in this chapter to mediate between the internal and the external realms. The arc of awareness, in other words, is postulated to be the instrument through which an external reality is translated into an internal conceptual awareness.

The supposition that some such instrument of cognition is indispensable has been a basic component of every philosophical system of significance. Philosopher E.F. Schumacher describes this postulate as "the Great Truth of '*adaequatio*' ": "Nothing can be known without there being an appropriate 'instrument' in the makeup of the knower. This is the Great Truth of '*adaequatio*' (adequateness), which defines knowledge as *adaequatio rei et intellectus*—the understanding of the knower must be adequate to the thing to be known" (Schumacher, 1977, p. 39).

This philosophical precept is perhaps best illustrated by reference to the limitations on our faculties of sensory perception. The human auditory and visual senses, for example, are extremely limited with respect to the spectra of wavelengths that are perceptible. Those wavelengths that fall outside of the perceptible spectra can be perceived only after they have been translated into stimuli to which our organic "instruments" of sensory perception are receptive.

The application of the concept of *adaequatio* to cognition itself, however, is far more profound. The "instrument" of cognition within the human "knower" is hypothesized to be the hyperneuronal arc of awareness. Cognition, therefore, is destined to be a reflection of the binary code of that instrument. The two-process model of information coding within the hyperneuronal arc applies to all sensory input. If information exists in the phenomenal universe that is not susceptible to coding within the binary processes of the hyperneuronal arc, then it is simply neither perceivable nor cognizable.

The hyperneuronal arc of awareness therefore is conceived to be the instrument of *adaequatio* necessary for cognition of a phenomenal universe of matter and energy in space and time. The cognition of the dimension of time requires some physiological process in time, and that process is manifest in the impulse frequency, or the internal focus, of the arc of awareness. Similarly, the cognition of the dimensions of space requires some physiological process in space, and that process is manifest in the spatial conformation, or the external focus, of the arc of awareness. And ultimately, within every episode of conceptual awareness, time is cognizable relative to space, and space is cognizable relative to time. Together, space and time arise in awareness as conceptualizations involving their correlative properties—matter and energy. In essence, therefore, the terms of *adaequatio* fusing the internal realm of conscious awareness with the external domain of physical reality are the three dimensions of space and the dimension of time: the senses of the mind. Out of these senses the entire phenomenal universe of matter and energy arises in conceptual awareness.

A Physiological Model of Mind

If the brain was so simple we could understand it, we would be so simple that we couldn't.

Lyall Watson

The Physiological Model of Mind, therefore, proposes that each episode of subjective awareness is a function of the focusing of neuronal conduction within a particular transcortical electrochemical arc. There are two intimately related parameters to this focusing of the hyperneuronal arc. First, the hyperneuronal arc must reflect an external focus involving the conformation of the arc within the three dimensions of physical brain space. Second, the hyperneuronal arc must reflect an internal focus involving the frequency of neuronal conduction along the path of the hyperneuronal arc's external focus. In the Physiological Model of Mind, the two parameters of focus to the hyperneuronal arc of awareness define

both a specific state and the operations within that state. Subjective awareness, then, is determined by essentially the same binary coding system
that was demonstrated to coordinate complex motor performances
through neuronal conduction to the contractile systems peripheral to the
brain. The external focus of the hyperneuronal arc within the three dimensions of brain space determines the specificity of the hyperneuronal arc
of awareness. The internal focus of the hyperneuronal arc, on the other
hand, determines the intensity of that arc. The mechanisms for encoding information within the hyperneuronal arc of awareness, then, are
limited to variations within the specificity and intensity of focus. This
binary model of coding provides a vast capacity for code variation. The
capacity for code variation, in turn, determines the volume of information that can be encoded.

The recognition that the brain employs a binary method of encoding
subjective awareness has profound implications for the nature of human
cognition. If the brain is limited to encoding conceptual awareness exclusively through the specificity and intensity of the focus of the hyperneuronal arc of awareness, conceptualization and cognition ultimately will
be limited to a corresponding binary modality. This proposition embodies
Schumacher's philosophical "truth" of *adaequatio*, which postulates that
"nothing can be known without there being an appropriate instrument
in the makeup of the knower." In short, the very terms of cognition are
defined and limited by the binary processes of coding. Because the
processes of thought are binary, thought itself is binary.

Cognition, of course, is a manifestation of subjective awareness, and
subjective awareness arises in consciousness only as conceptualization.
Concepts, in other words, are the fundamental elements of cognition.
The Physiological Model of Mind hypothesizes that each conceptualization that arises in subjective awareness is determined by the internal and
the external focuses of the hyperneuronal arc associated with that episode of awareness. The spatial conformation of the hyperneuronal arc
delimits the corresponding concept within the dimensions of space. The
frequency of the hyperneuronal arc delimits the corresponding concept
within the dimension of time. Each concept that arises in subjective awareness reflects a synthesis of these spatial and temporal delimitations. The
limits, in other words, define the concept. The concept of "matter" arises
to describe conceptual objects localized in space, whereas the concept of
"energy" arises to describe conceptual processes involving the transformations of conceptual objects over time. The realm of conceptual cognition, therefore, is limited to the conceptual terms of matter and energy
in space and time. These, in fact, are the fundamental terms of cognition
on which Western empiricism is grounded.

The Physiological Model of Mind, moreover, is essentially mechanistic
and deterministic. Learning is understood to occur within the Physiological Model of Mind in substantially the same way that it was perceived

to occur within the contractile and the energy systems. In other words, organic adaptations within the physiological processes of the brain provide a plausible explanation for even the most profound episodes of learning. Sophisticated systems of regulation and coordination can be hypothesized to occur on a strictly mechanistic and deterministic basis without resort to any explanations involving a faculty of mind that is separate from the deterministic physiological processes of the central nervous system. The Physiological Model of Mind is therefore based on the apparently mechanistic processes that transpire at the cellular, molecular, and atomic levels. These electrochemical processes are understood to be the substrate of consciousness.

Although it appears certain that the rule of specificity of practice and the rule of intensity of practice apply to the mechanistic processes of learning even within the framework of the Physiological Model of Mind, that model is lacking the fundamental agency that distinguishes practice from experience: the willpower of the mind. If the will cannot be found lurking within the hyperneuronal arcs of awareness or even within the microsystems that are the constituent elements of those hyperneuronal arcs, perhaps it will be found at the next deeper level of analysis, to which these writings progress in chapter 6, in pursuit of an Empirical Model of the Phenomenal Universe.

This chapter, then, has conceived an extensive, though highly speculative and still incomplete, Physiological Model of Mind. Such a model seems relatively unobjectionable in explaining most of the functions of the brain, including many functions associated with consciousness. Physiological processes of permanent and semipermanent facilitation of neuronal conduction—most notably the processes categorized as memory—can be understood to provide a "self-programming" mechanism for the brain's organic machinery of regulation and coordination. Thought becomes, then, in the words of physicist and philosopher David Bohm, "the active response of memory in every phase of life." Bohm goes on to emphasize the mechanical nature of thought:

> It is clear that thought, considered in this way as the response of memory, is basically mechanical in its order of operation. Either it is a repetition of some previously existent structure drawn from memory, or else it is some combination arrangement and organization of these memories into further structures of ideas and concepts, categories, etc. These combinations may possess a certain kind of novelty resulting from the fortuitous interplay of elements of memory, but it is clear that such novelty is still essentially mechanical (like the new combinations appearing in a kaleidoscope) (Bohm, 1983, pp. 50-51).

The idea that all consciousness is strictly the result of mechanical physiological processes is, however, far less palatable than is the lesser admission that some or even most processes of consciousness are entirely mechanical. Bohm, for example, exempts the "original and unconditioned response of intelligence" from the mechanical determinism of processes of "thought." Such an exemption, of course, has far-reaching consequences:

> *If intelligence is to be an unconditioned act of perception, its ground cannot be in structures such as cells, molecules, atoms, elementary particles, etc. Ultimately, anything that is determined by the laws of such structures must be in the field of what can be known, i.e., stored up in memory, and thus it will have to have the mechanical nature of anything that can be assimilated in the basically mechanical character of the process of thought. The actual operation of intelligence is thus beyond the possibility of being determined or conditioned by factors that can be included in any knowable law. So, we see that the ground of intelligence must be in the undetermined and unknown flux, that is also the ground of all definable forms of matter. Intelligence is thus not deducible or explainable on the basis of any branch of knowledge (e.g., physics or biology). Its origin is deeper and more inward than any knowable order that could describe it. (Indeed, it has to comprehend the very order of definable forms of matter through which we would hope to comprehend intelligence.)* (Bohm, 1983, pp. 51-52).

Bohm, then, conceives of intelligence as arising from the "undetermined and unknown flux, that is also the ground of all definable forms of matter." The question of whether this retreat from a Physiological Model of Mind grounded in mechanistic determinism constitutes a wholesale abandonment of understanding or instead the removal of understanding to a new and deeper level can be answered only by an analysis of that "universal flux" from which the phenomenal universe, including the brain and intelligent consciousness, are conceived to arise.

Note

[1]The Physiological Model of Mind developed in this chapter draws upon the research and theories of many prominent neuroscientists. Chapter 5 presents a relatively technical summary of the prevailing conceptions of brain structure and function, together with a brief review of several of the more powerful and interesting theories concerning the physiology of subjective awareness. The reader is referred to chapter 5 for clarification and elaboration of the scientific data on which the Physiological Model of Mind is grounded. However, it should be noted that the Physiological Model of Mind developed in the body of this chapter goes well beyond the characteristically restrained hypotheses and modelings of brain functions found in the neuroscientific literature.

5

A Physiological Model of Mind: The Evidence

Thoughts without contents are empty, intuitions without concepts are blind.

Immanuel Kant

The nervous system consists of the central nervous system, which includes the brain and the spinal cord, and the peripheral nervous system, which includes all other neuronal processes extending throughout the body. The primary functional unit of the nervous system is the neuron, which conducts the electrochemical action potentials, or neuronal impulses, which integrate the billions of nerve cells within the peripheral and the central nervous systems. Each nerve cell, or neuron, is comprised of a cell body, out of which extend multiple short branches called dendrites, and of one longer neuronal extension called the axon. Axons vary in length from barely distinguishable to over 1 meter.

Figure 6 is a diagram of a typical neuron, drawn to scale and enlarged approximately 250 times. Nerve impulses are conveyed from the cell body through the axon and into the neuron's terminal fibers. The axon depicted (which is folded for schematic purposes) would be one centimeter long in actual size. Many axons, such as the one shown in this figure, are insulated by a myelin sheath, broken at periodic intervals by nodes of Ranvier.

Information transfer between individual nerve cells occurs at cell junctions called synapses. The predominant type of synapse involves the synaptic junction of the axon of one neuron and the dendrites of a second neuron. However, synaptic junctions can exist also between the axons

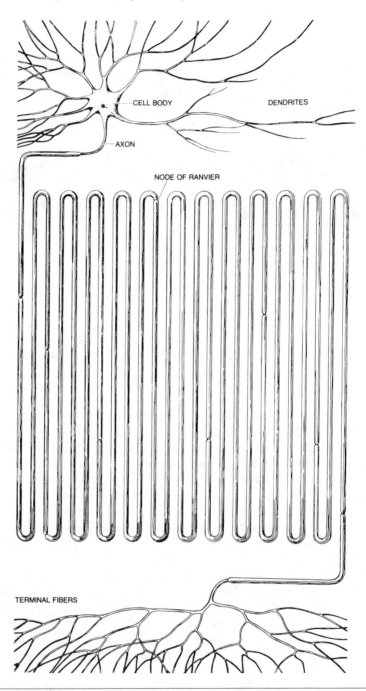

Figure 6.   A diagram of a typical neuron. *Note.* From ''The Neuron'' (p. 56) by C.F. Stevens. Copyright © 1979 by Scientific American, Inc. All rights reserved.

of two neurons, between the dendrites of two neurons, and between the axon or dendrites of one neuron and the cell body of a second neuron.

The neural network is extremely complicated and multifaceted. Most neurons possess a multitude of synaptic junctions, numbering in the thousands. Moreover, these synapses usually join the neuron to numerous other neurons, both proximate and distant. It is not uncommon for a single neuron to be linked directly in a conduction network to more than 1,000 other neurons; occasionally this number can reach to over 10,000.

The most common process of neuronal conduction proceeds in the following way. Incoming or afferent nerve impulses are received by the neuron at synaptic junctions located on the cell body and proximate dendritic processes. The incoming impulses, which can be either excitatory or inhibitory, are screened and integrated by mechanisms principally within the surface membrane of the nerve cell, and output messages, if any, are then passed from the junction of the cell body and its axonal extension outward along the axon. The axon, therefore, is the primary outgoing, or efferent, channel for each individual nerve cell. The axons of the larger nerves are enveloped in a myelin sheath, which appears to function primarily as an insulation for the cylindrical membrane of the axon, permitting electrical conduction along the axon with greater efficiency. Nodal interruptions in the myelin sheath occur approximately at each millimeter, bringing the axonal membrane into close apposition with the extracellular fluid necessary for generation of the neuronal action potential. As a consequence, nerve impulses exhibit a process of saltatory transmission, in which the action potential generated at one node alters the electrical conformation of the axonal membrane at the next node, causing the nerve impulse to appear to jump from node to node along the axon. The nerve cells are embedded in glial cells, which appear to serve critically important structural, developmental, insulative, and nutritive functions in support of the network of neurons.

As a first approximation, the organization of the nervous system can be understood to consist of a system of afferent conduction leading from peripheral sensory receptors[1] throughout the body into the central nervous system, and of a system of efferent impulses directed from the central nervous system into peripheral areas throughout the body. Afferent impulses therefore give rise to sensory perception, whereas efferent impulses are responsible for executive functions such as regulation and movement. In addition, the peripheral nervous system contains (distributed throughout the body) nerve cell concentrations, called autonomic ganglia, which, through their afferent and efferent connections, serve to regulate many of the body's automatic functions, especially those involving the internal organs and systems.

The Action Potential

The propagation of the nerve impulse is due to a process involving two aspects. First, the electrical conduction or cable property of the axon permits an electrical charge to be conducted a short distance along the axon. Second, an electrochemical change across the axon's membrane in response to the short-lived electrical conduction causes the propagation of a full neuronal impulse, or action potential. Strict electrical conduction, without the propagation of an action potential, is not adequate to explain neuronal transmission. Rather, the electrical conduction that precedes the action potential along the axon appears to be amplified and coded for propagation by the electrochemical processes of the action potential.

In its resting, or inactive, state, a neuron possesses an internal environment that is approximately 70 millivolts negative compared to the external cell environment. Ordinarily, the cell membrane would be sufficiently permeable to potassium and sodium ions to enable their concentrations to stabilize at an electrical equilibrium level through exchanges across the cell membrane. To prevent equalization of electrical charge across the neuronal membrane, thereby maintaining a substantial electrical potential across that membrane, each neuron's membrane contains a multitude of sodium-potassium ATPase pumps. These molecular active transport mechanisms are complex protein molecules embedded in the axonal membrane that utilize the energy captured from the reduction of ATP to ADP to fuel an exchange for each pump of approximately 200 sodium ions for 130 potassium ions across the cell membrane every second. Even a small neuron will contain on the order of a million such pumps. As a result of the action of these membrane pumps, there is a concentration of positively charged potassium ions that is 10 times greater inside the neuron than outside and a concentration of positively charged sodium ions 10 times greater outside the neuron than inside. In its resting state, the axonal membrane is readily permeable to potassium ions but virtually impermeable to sodium ions. Therefore, there is a net potassium ion flow from within the axon outward and no countervailing influx of sodium ions. The consequent net deficiency of positive ions within the membrane relative to the outside of the membrane results in an internal axonal voltage that is approximately 70 millivolts negative compared to the external environment (see Figure 7).

The electrical charge that precedes the action potential for short distances along the nerve axon increases the permeability of the cell membrane to sodium ions. The mechanism for this increase involves the opening of "voltage-gated" sodium channels in the axonal membrane in response to the slight decrease in the 70-millivolt differential across the membrane. The key to the propagation of an action potential therefore involves the fact that sodium conductance across the cell membrane is a function of the membrane potential. In other words, as the resting potential of the axonal membrane—approximately -70 millivolts—is lowered, the rate of sodium conductance across the membrane increases.

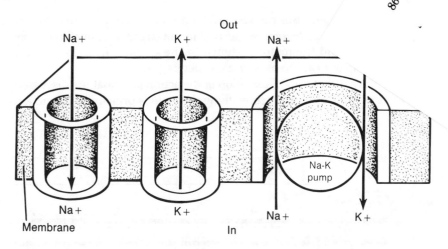

Figure 7. A schematic diagram of the three primary mechanisms involved in the propagation of the nerve impulse: the sodium (Na+) channel, the potassium (K+) channel, and the adenosine triphosphatase pump, or ATP pump (Na-K pump). The "passive" sodium and potassium channels are "voltage-gated." *Note.* Reprinted by permission of the publisher from *Principles of Neural Science* (p. 33), edited by E.R. Kandel and J.H. Swartz. Copyright © 1985 by Elsevier Science Publishing Co., Inc.

The process becomes self-reinforcing at approximately −40 millivolts— the "action threshold"—as the conductance of sodium ions into the neuron lowers the membrane potential, which further increases the membrane permeability to sodium, which further lowers the membrane potential. The opening of the voltage-gated sodium channels is sustained, and the membrane potential jumps from −40 millivolts to +40 millivolts with extreme rapidity. This superthreshold change in membrane potential is the action potential. As the internal cell environment becomes positively charged with respect to the external environment, the sodium channels in the membrane close and potassium ion channels in the membrane open, greatly increasing potassium conductance across the membrane. This results in the return of the axon to a negative internal electrical potential.

The peak positive membrane potential reflected in a neuronal impulse is therefore approximately +40 millivolts. The ATP pumps, assisted by the closing of the sodium ion channels and the opening of the potassium ion channels, restore the resting membrane potential of −70 millivolts during a brief but rate-limiting "refractory" period following each action potential. This system of sodium-potassium ion exchange is efficient and rapid enough, however, to permit nerves to generate on the order of everal hundred impulses per second. Conduction along the nerve axon can be as rapid as 100 meters per second in the largest myelinated nerves of the sensory and the motor systems. In the smallest fibers, however, conduction speed can be as low as 3 meters per second.

Figure 8 is a diagramatic illustration of the action potential. As discussed above, nerve impulse conduction along the axon is principally a function

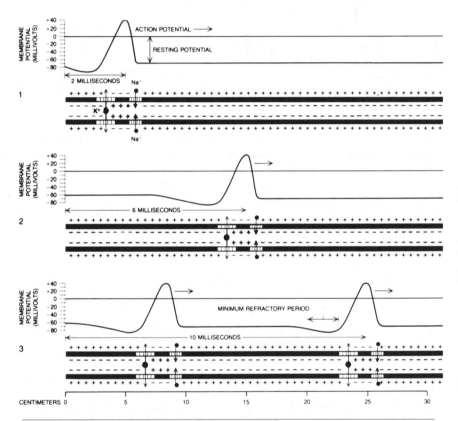

Figure 8. A diagramatic illustration of the action potential. *Note.* From "The Neuron" (p. 20) by C.F. Stevens. Copyright © 1979 by Scientific American, Inc. All rights reserved.

of a localized inflow of sodium ions (Na+) and a localized outflow of potassium ions (K+) through "voltage gated" channels in the axon membrane. The impulse originates in a neuron as a result of a slight depolarization, or decrease, in the negative potential of the neuronal membrane (most commonly as the result of the postsynaptic action of neurotransmitters). This slight change of the electrical potential across the axonal membrane opens sodium channels in that membrane, further altering the voltage and thereby opening additional sodium channels, until the inner membrane voltage is locally positive. This voltage reversal closes the sodium channels and opens potassium channels, and the resulting outflow of potassium ions rapidly restores the negative membrane potential. This microsystemic dynamic, called the action potential, propagates itself along the axon (1,2), and can be followed by another action potential after a brief "refractory" period (3). The speed of impulse propagation indicated in the diagrams is based on measurements of conduction speed in the giant axon of the squid.

Because the electrical profiles of the action potentials do not appear to vary measurably among the multitude of neurons, conduction of the action potential along the axon is presumed to be coded in patterns of impulse. These patterns vary in frequency, up to the rate limitation of the refractory period, and in rhythm. Rhythm refers to patterns of frequency variation over time. Subtle variations in impulse amplitude also are conceivable, although researchers have not found measurable evidence for such a modality of neuronal coding.

Synaptic Transmission

The process of neuronal impulse conduction across the synaptic gaps that separate successive neurons from one another differs markedly from the electrochemical mechanism for propagation of the action potential. The action potential is conveyed across the synaptic gap by chemical agents that are released from the presynaptic membrane in response to an action potential in the presynaptic axon. When a neuronal impulse reaches the knoblike presynaptic axonal terminal, voltage-gated calcium channels in the axonal membrane open, allowing the influx of free calcium into the presynaptic region of the axon. The calcium influx apparently triggers the perfusion of a specific chemical agent from the presynaptic axon into the synaptic gap. This chemical transmitter diffuses across the synaptic gap to react electrochemically with receptive regions on the postsynaptic cell membrane. The most prevalent mode of postsynaptic cell response to neurotransmitters involves alterations of the permeability of the postsynaptic membrane to sodium and potassium ions, triggering the propagation of an action potential within the postsynaptic neuron when the action threshold potential across the postsynaptic cell membrane is reached. Membrane channels in the postsynaptic neuron, such as the synaptic sodium and potassium channels, are activated by chemical reactions involving the neurotransmitter. These channels are therefore understood to be "chemically gated" rather than voltage gated.

Figure 9 depicts the vesicular hypothesis of synaptic conduction involving the release and uptake of the neurotransmitter acetylcholine.

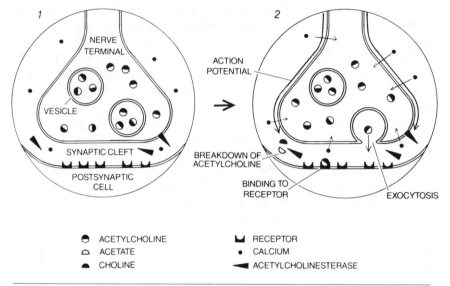

Figure 9.   A schematic diagram of the vesicular hypothesis of synaptic conduction. *Note.* From "The Release of Acetylcholine" (p. 60) by Y. Dunant and M. Israel. Copyright © 1979 by Scientific American, Inc. All rights reserved.

Approximately half of the acetylcholine in the presynaptic terminal is stored in vesicles when the neuron is at rest (1). The arrival of an action potential at the presynaptic terminal causes an influx of calcium ions into the presynaptic terminal. The calcium ions are hypothesized to cause the vesicles to fuse with the presynaptic membrane in such a way that the contents of the vesicles are perfused into the synaptic cleft. Synaptic transmission is accomplished by the attachment of molecules of acetylcholine to receptive sites located on the postsynaptic membrane. The acetylcholine is then broken down into choline and acetate by the enzyme acetylcholinesterase, found in the synaptic cleft (2). Recently, researchers have suggested an alternative cytoplasmic hypothesis of synaptic conduction, in which the presynaptic vesicles play a slightly different role.

Until recently, it was believed that a particular presynaptic terminal will release a single characteristic type of chemical transmitter tailored to combine with proximate receptive regions on the postsynaptic membrane to achieve a specific gating effect. Now, however, it has been revealed that many neurons employ as many as three different neurotransmitters, or "cotransmitters," that are believed to act synergistically. Overall, researchers have identified more than 50 distinct neurotransmitters. Some of these are amines or amino acids, but the majority are compound amino acid configurations called peptides. Interestingly, many of these neurotransmitters also act as hormones. Each distinct neurotransmitter apparently triggers a characteristic gating effect when it reacts with a particular receptive molecule embedded in the postsynaptic membrane. Some transmitters open sodium and potassium channels indiscriminately, whereas others exhibit high degrees of selectivity in their gating effects. The chemical-gating effect resulting from the interaction of a particular transmitter with the postsynaptic membrane therefore can be either excitatory—that is, lowering or depolarizing the membrane potential, thereby increasing the likelihood that an action potential will result—or inhibitory—that is, raising or hyperpolarizing the membrane potential, thereby decreasing the likelihood that an action potential will result.

The membrane of the nerve cell body differs substantially from the membrane of the nerve cell axon. The axonal membrane appears to function through gating mechanisms that control ionic currents of sodium, potassium, and calcium. The membrane of the nerve cell body, however, exhibits a greater selection of gating mechanisms that generate as many as seven distinct ionic currents. Variations in cell body membrane function provide a physiological basis for individualization and functional specialization among nerve cells.

Synaptic conduction, therefore, differs entirely from axonal conduction in the methods of coding and transmission. The action pattern at synapses reflects two important phenomena: temporal summation and spatial summation. Temporal summation involves an immediate summing effect as the concentration of neurotransmitter increases within the synaptic gap. The greater the frequency of the presynaptic neuronal impulse, the greater will be the concentration of transmitter released into the synaptic gap. The greater this concentration, in turn, the greater will be the postsynaptic effect resulting from chemical gating. Spatial summation involves a subthreshold integration of excitatory and inhibitory impulses that converge within the synaptic gap. The integration occurs by subthreshold alterations in the postsynaptic membrane potential caused by the combined action of the synaptic transmitters.

Until recently, it was believed that transmission of neuronal impulses across synaptic gaps was exclusively a chemical process not involving significant electrical conduction. However, researchers have discovered evidence of interneuronal electrical conduction through the frequently dense dendritic processes that branch out from the nerve cell bodies. This evidence suggests the likelihood that transmission between nerve cells can occur through electrical conduction through and between dendrites, in addition to chemical transmission across synapses. Nerve cell junctions that do not exhibit characteristic synaptic mechanisms of neurotransmission are referred to as ephaptic junctions.

Not only do the synaptic and ephaptic junctions between neurons contain mechanisms for highly sophisticated processing of neuronal impulses, but recent investigations also have demonstrated the existence of a "second-messenger" system for processing neuronal information. Interestingly, the existence of such secondary transmitters was first discovered during the investigation of the breakdown of glycogen into glucose within the cells of the liver. The hormone adrenalin, which previously had been believed to be the agent of this chemical change, was found to stimulate the liver cell membrane to release within the cell a second substance that actually caused the reduction of hepatic glycogen. A similar two-step process was later found to exist in some, but not all, synaptic transmissions as well. Accordingly, neurotransmitters are now understood to operate not only through their chemical gating effect on the polarization of the postsynaptic membrane but also by triggering the activity of a second chemical that works its effect within the postsynaptic cell. Second-messenger systems have been hypothesized as the mechanism for the structural adaptations that arise in consciousness as long- and short-term memory and for various other more or less durable structural adaptations of functional significance to the neuron.

The processes involved in neuronal transmission, then, are extremely sophisticated subcellular microsystems that permit a virtually unlimited range of informational coding and impulse processing. The molecular model of neuronal coding for axonal conduction exhibits a capacity for transmission of a potentially infinite range of information employing as code terms the frequency and rhythm of the action potentials propagated. Similarly, the molecular model of synaptic transmission of neuronal impulses reflects an unlimited coding capability based on variable types and concentrations of chemical neurotransmitters and on subtle shadings of electrical conduction through dendritic processes. The microsystems of axonal impulse propagation and synaptic and ephaptic junctional processing combine to create a macrosystem of neuronal conduction through which all neural functions are presumed to transpire.

The Autonomic Nervous System

The neural framework throughout the body—that is, the neural macrosystem—is largely determined by genetic decree and therefore reflects patterns of neuronal conduction supportive to individual and species survival within the evolutionary process of natural selection. A human possesses at birth a highly sophisticated system of neuronal conduction that maintains and regulates the extraordinary mechanisms that sustain the basic life functions. Regulation of such critical, sophisticated functions as blood glucose level, water metabolism, body temperature, circulation, respiration, digestion, reproduction, and basic sensory-motor response are accomplished through built-in patterns of neuronal conduction. Most of these functions are assumed to manifest initially without awareness—that is, without either conscious volition or attention. They are instead mechanical processes of the body that are remote from the awareness of mind and encoded structurally within the framework of neuronal conduction.

Basic homeostasis, which involves maintenance of a dynamic equilibrium within the electrochemical processes that constitute the internal environment of the physical body, including metabolic and hormonal functions, is governed principally through the autonomic nervous system. The autonomic nervous system is comprised of two anatomically and physiologically distinct systems that work in complementary opposition to each other.

The sympathetic autonomic nervous system operates either directly or through the agency of hormonal secretions from the endocrine system and appears controlled from brain centers in the hypothalamus. The sympathetic system, mediated by the neurotransmitter norepinephrine, accelerates bodily functions, apparently to prepare the individual for intensive or protractive activity. Among the effects of excitation from the sympathetic system are the acceleration of the heart rate, the selective dilation and constriction of veins and arteries, the dilation of the bronchi, the slowing of peristalsis, and the dilation of the pupils.

The parasympathetic autonomic nervous system, on the other hand, operates to maintain autonomic processes at normal homeostatic equilibrium, in contravention of the effects of the sympathetic system. It employs the neurotransmitter acetylcholine, or ACh, instead of norepinephrine, and systemic control appears centered in the midbrain, pons, and medulla. Excitation of the parasympathetic system generally reverses the effects of the sympathetic system, thereby returning the internal environment to a condition of homeostasis.

Working in concert, these two systems maintain a dynamic equilibrium within the autonomic processes of the body despite potentially dramatic variations in stimuli from external sources.

Anatomically, the parasympathetic and the sympathetic autonomic systems are insinuated within the cranial and spinal nerve pathways that emerge from the central nervous system. The autonomic neural processes, however, involve a number of peripheral ganglionic junctions of neuronal nuclei that appear to be processing centers that interrupt linear pathways of neuronal conduction. Consequently, much of the regulation and control of autonomic functions occurs reflexively in neuronal ganglia remote from the central nervous system. Ultimately, however, autonomic functions appear to be regulated and coordinated through mechanisms centered deep within the brain, primarily localized in the vicinity of the ''midline ventricular system of the brain stem.'' Neuropsychologist and neurosurgeon Karl Pribram has suggested that the structures involved in autonomic regulation are actually specialized sensory receptors that "function as 'state' sensitive elements of a variety of servomechanisms—christened 'homeostats' by Cannon (1929)—concerned with the regulation of appetitive-consummatory functions" (Pribram, 1981, pp. 174-175). Whatever the specific mechanisms of brain regulation involved in the basic metabolic and hormonal processes, it is clear that they are genetically built-in and remote from both volitional and attentive awareness. It should be emphasized, however, that such autonomic processes are not entirely inaccessible to conscious observation or control.

Not all acts of body and mind, of course, are structurally encoded at birth. Throughout an individual's life, constant adaptations and elaborations of the innate neural macrosystem are presumed to occur, affecting even the autonomic functions.

At some early point in the life cycle of an individual, the patterns of neural activity are presumed to produce both automatic motor response and the phenomenon of mind as manifest in the subjective experience of awareness. The mind, of course, is believed to be centered within the brain. Yet ultimately, it is the mind that believes and presumes, investigates and analyzes, and distinguishes its own conscious functions from those brain functions it characterizes as automatic and autonomic.

The Brain

In evolutionary terms, the newest part of the brain is the telencephalon, which is composed of the large, convoluted cerebral hemispheres. The telencephalon blossoms out of the diencephalon, which is also called the old brain or the higher brainstem. The third and fourth anatomical divisions are the mesencephalon, or midbrain, and the rhombencephalon, or hindbrain.

The rhombencephalon and mesencephalon include the upper swelling of the spinal cord, the reticular formation, the cerebellum, the medulla and pons, and the superior and inferior colliculi. Many of the mechanisms for regulating and coordinating the autonomic nervous system are centered in this region. It is the only part of the brain not incapacitated by the electrical hyperactivity that occurs during grand mal epileptic seizures. Nearly all afferent neuronal conduction passes through and is potentially processed by these lower-brain centers.

The diencephalon consists of those brain areas intervening between the cerebral hemispheres of the telencephalon and the lower-brain centers of the rhombencephalon and mesencephalon. The most notable anatomical landmarks within the diencephalon include the thalamus, the hypothalamus, the subthalamic nucleus, the septum, the third ventricle, and the pituitary glandular complex. The diencephalon appears to be a critical processing center for almost all neuronal conduction, both afferent and efferent, involving the telencephalon. Diencephalic cellular interrupts therefore appear to be centrally implicated in virtually all complex sensory and motor functions.

The thalamic nuclei within the diencephalon blossom into the two hemispheres of the telencephalon. The most prominent feature of the telencephalon is the highly convoluted, gray mass of nerve cell nuclei that constitutes the cerebral cortex, or neocortex. The topography of the cortex is described in terms of convolutions or hills, called gyri, and furrows or valleys, called sulci. The deepest sulci within the cortex are termed fissures. The geography of the cortex is not well delineated, but divisions have been drawn in correspondence with the enveloping cranial bones: the occipital, the temporal, the parietal, and the frontal regions. Located beneath the neocortical gray matter that blankets the telencephalon are a multitude of axonal nerve tracts constituting the white matter of the cerebrum. The telencephalon also contains critically important subcortical areas that lie at the base of the cerebral hemispheres in close proximity to the diencephalon. These include the hippocampus, the amygdalas, the olfactory fields, and the corpus striatum, or basal ganglia. Within the corpus striatum are two distinct cell groupings termed the globus pallidus and the striatum. The striatum in turn contains the caudate nucleus and the putamen.

The telencephalon appears to be the principal locus of the higher-brain functions involved in conceptualization and memory and also is centrally implicated in complex sensory and motor activity and emotional response. Without question, the telencephalon is indispensable to the subjective experience of conscious awareness and to most compound automatic functions as well (see Figure 10).

Despite the identification of these many anatomically distinct cell groupings within the brain, researchers are only beginning to correlate specific, discrete functions to particular cell ensembles. Most instances of higher-brain function involve systems of neuronal conduction that implicate numerous anatomical areas. These pathways of neuronal conduction, however, are so complex and diffuse that discernment of the functional relationship between anatomical areas is often speculative. Contemporary models of brain physiology, therefore, remain largely inchoate and approximate.

Traditionally, the physiological model of the brain has presumed that the basic agency or mechanism of brain function is the neuron; and neuronal activity within the brain has been understood to be governed by essentially the same processes that apply to impulse conduction within the peripheral nervous system. The interplay of electrochemical action potentials along neuronal axons, together with neurotransmission across

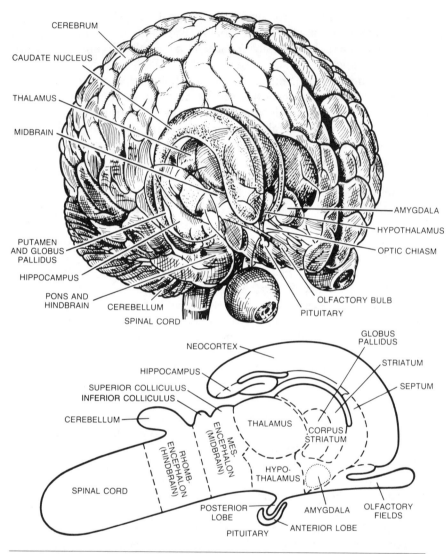

Figure 10.   The major anatomical landmarks of the brain and brain stem. The top diagram shows an artificial transparency of the exterior regions of the brain so that certain internal structures can be portrayed. The bottom diagram is a highly schematic depiction of the mammalian brain and spinal cord. *Note.* From "The Organization of the Brain" (p. 102) by W.J.H. Nauta and M. Feirtag. Copyright © 1979 by Scientific American, Inc. All rights reserved.

synaptic and ephaptic junctions, are therefore presumed to be the predominant mechanisms of brain function.

Much of the basal metabolism of the body is utilized to maintain the ATP sodium-potassium pumps that set each neuron into a state of electrochemical resonance. The ATP is derived from the oxidative metabolism of blood glucose. Consequently, the brain utilizes approximately 20% of the oxygen assimilated by the body at rest. Not only does this neuronal resonance itself create discernible electrical potentials within the brain, but it is the necessary precondition to neuronal conduction of any kind.

One of the most provocative features of brain activity involves the seemingly "spontaneous" generation of neuronal impulses by neurons within the brain. French neurophysiologist Jean-Pierre Changeux elaborates:

> *The electroencephalogram clearly shows that even during sleep, the cerebral cortex produces intense electrical activity. A microelectrode in any cortical nerve cell shows that there is spontaneous generation of electrical impulses. This phenomenon is generalized. Even neurons in tissue culture, such as those derived from a tumor like a neuroblastoma, produce spontaneous action potentials. The analysis of these impulse generators has been facilitated by the remarkable temporal regularity of the impulses. They act as oscillators.* (Changeux, 1985, p. 77)

Changeux hypothesizes a molecular model—involving "four molecular channels, three ions, two pumps, and ATP"—that provides a mechanical explanation for neuronal oscillators. Accordingly, Changeux actually rejects the notion that neuronal impulses arise "spontaneously" within the brain, although he emphasizes that many neuronal oscillators are tuned to operate as "stochastic, or random, impulse generators" (Changeux, 1985, p. 81).

The electrochemical resonance of the brain, therefore, is a combination of basal tonus and neuronal impulse conduction—both afferent conduction entering the brain and conduction originating "spontaneously" within the brain—and this resonance can be crudely registered and measured through electroencephalography (EEG). Brain-wave activity exhibits distinctive patterns that correlate with various states of consciousness or unconsciousness. For example, the electrical patterns of brain activity differ dramatically between sleep and wakefulness. The principal distinction appears to involve the pattern and perhaps the intensity of afferent neuronal impulses transmitted into the cortical areas of the brain from the lower-brain centers.

The Reticular Formation

The reticular formation, located within the brainstem and extending through the medulla and pons to the base of the thalamus and hypothalamus, is a network of short-process neurons that have been demonstrated to activate the cortical tone that corresponds to wakeful brain activity.

The reticular formation has been identified as possessing both ascending and descending aspects, each with apparently distinct functions. The afferent sensory nerves interface with the ascending reticular formation through brushlike interconnections. Apparently, when afferent impulses reach a threshold level of intensity (which seems capable of being preset, or "biased," for sensitivity and specificity), the ascending reticular process relays electrochemical impulses throughout the cortex, thereby creating a cortical tone corresponding to wakefulness. This cortical tone appears indispensable to the functioning of the cortex, as if by generalized electrical stimulation the cortex is awakened and sensitized for the receipt and processing of afferent impulses. Wakefulness is not possible when the reticular formation is destroyed or severely damaged. It is hypothesized that the collateral connections between the afferent sensory impulses and the reticular formation provide a mode of inhibition or enhancement of sensory input modulated by neuronal feedback from the thalamic or cortical areas of the higher brain.

The descending reticular formation interfaces with efferent impulses through similar brushlike interconnections. Damage to the descending reticular formation leads to jerkiness and impaired coordination in motor response, suggesting that the descending reticular formation has some regulating or integrating function with respect to the efferent motor conduction.

The upper areas of the reticular formation appear to have facilitative effects on both afferent and efferent impulses, whereas the lower portions of the formation exhibit inhibitory effects.

It appears that the level of cortical tone is substantially modulated by action of the reticular formation and that greater or lesser levels of cortical arousal have dramatic effects on personality and behavior. The reticular formation also appears to be substantially involved in regulation of the autonomic nervous system.

The reticular formation is, then, a primary processing center located principally within the rhombencephalon and mesencephalon. Most, but not all, afferent and efferent conduction appears to be affected by its operation. Moreover, it is indispensable to consciousness. Yet there are indications that the functioning of the reticular formation is controlled substantially by higher-brain centers. At the very least, it is clear that most efferent and afferent conduction is subject to multiple levels of processing in addition to reticular processing.

The Diencephalic Interrupt

At the top of the reticular formation, located in the heart of the diencephalon, is another major cellular interrupt, or neuronal processing center: the thalamus. This center appears to operate as the gateway to the telencephalon. Virtually all higher-brain functions, whether automatic or voluntary, appear to involve conduction through this diencephalic processing center.

The thalamus receives afferent impulses from all the sensoria (except olfaction) through the spinothalamic tract, the medial lemniscus, fibers from the inferior and the superior colliculi, and the optic tracts. The thalamic nuclei, on which these sensory inputs are entrained, project neuronal pathways to specific sensory areas of the cortex. The thalamus, therefore, appears to be a final processing center for all sensory conduction entering the telencephalon, with the apparent exception of olfaction. The projections from the thalamus to the sensory cortex are reciprocated by projections returning from the sensory cortex to the thalamus.

The primary sensory areas of the cortex that receive the thalamocortical projections not only exhibit reciprocal vertical integration with the thalamus (through corticofugal tracts) but also display an extensive horizontal integration through nerve tracts that disperse throughout the neocortex. The wide expanses of neocortex traversed in this horizontal integration are called association areas and are presumed to be involved in the progressive processing of sensory input originating in the thalamocortical projections. Indeed, neurophysiologists Walle Nauta and Michael Feirtag have stated that "it is now known that the march of neural processing through the neocortex typically involves a sequence of association areas, and that a destination of the march seems invariably to be the hippocampus or the amygdala, or both" (Nauta & Feirtag, 1979, p. 49). Vertical integration between the thalamus and virtually all areas of the cortex, including the frontal and the temporal lobes, is achieved through the direct parallel tracts of the corona radiata.

The thalamus, in addition to the afferent sensory conduction it receives and processes, receives in its anterior portion major motoric projections from the subcortical area of the corpus striatum and from the cerebellum. Virtually all areas of the neocortex project without interruption to the corpus striatum, which, after several internal processing interrupts, projects through a major branch of the ansa lenticularis to the thalamus. In addition, extensive projections from throughout the neocortex descend to the pons, which in turn projects through major neural pathways to the cerebellum. The cerebellum, in turn, connects directly with the thalamus through the brachium conjunctivum. These motoric projections from the corpus striatum and the cerebellum are projected from the thalamus to the motor cortex of the telencephalon. The motor cortex not only reciprocates these projections from the thalamus but also projects to the reticular formation and even through the corticospinal tract directly to motor neurons within the spinal cord. There are, as well, efferent projections from other areas of the neocortex—that is, other than the motor cortex— that do not directly involve the thalamus but instead descend into regions of the rhombencephalon and mesencephalon, most notably the reticular formation.

This simplified description of the thalamic circuitry suggests the possibility that neural conduction either can be substantially limited to the projections between the thalamus and the sensory and motor areas of the neocortex or can implicate the vast neural network of the neocortex and the various subcortical processing centers. The physiological basis for the distinction between brain processes attended by conscious awareness and those characterized as automatic has been conjectured to rest upon this distinction between limited and extensive conductive processes. Processes of neural conduction limited to the sensory and the motor cortex areas can be hypothesized to transpire automatically without attendant awareness, whereas the integrated involvement of widespread cortical and subcortical regions can be hypothesized to trigger a subjective sense of conscious awareness.

Neurosurgeon Wilder Penfield identified the diencephalic gateways to these two alternative processing systems—one experienced as conscious awareness and the other as automatic—as the "conscious interpretive mechanism," or the "highest brain-mechanism," involving widespread cortical activity, and the "automatic sensory-motor mechanism," involving only areas of the sensory and motor cortex. Penfield suggested that petit mal automatism, a peculiar type of epilepsy, illustrates the distinction between these two mechanisms. This type of epileptic seizure is characterized by the departure of normal consciousness without the concurrent loss of automatic sensory-motor function. In fact, during a petit mal seizure exhibiting automatism, the sufferer can continue to execute even sophisticated automatic sensory-motor responses, notwithstanding the total departure of conscious awareness. However, automatism appears limited to the continuation of patterned responses already initiated and in progress and does not appear to permit new direction or initiative in response. Petit mal automatism is believed to be caused by localized electrical hyperactivity that incapacitates the diencephalic center that provides access to those widespread cerebral processes—especially those involving the temporal and the frontal lobes—attended by some degree of awareness. Petit mal epilepsy, however, does not interfere with the automatic processes that involve only the sensory and the motor cortices and that Penfield suggests are mediated through the automatic sensory-motor mechanism of the diencephalon:

> *The evidence from our studies of epileptic patterns suggests that gray matter in the highest brain mechanism has direct connection with these [evolutionarily recent] parts of the frontal and temporal lobes while the gray matter of the automatic sensory-motor mechanism is directly connected to the various areas of the sensory and motor cortex. One may assume that the highest brain mechanism makes its major connections with the sensory and motor cortex only through the automatic mechanism of the diencephalon (Penfield, 1975, p. 110).*

This distinction between a "conscious interpretive mechanism" and an "automatic sensory-motor mechanism" therefore is premised on the supposition that conscious awareness involves extensive, transcortical pathways of neuronal conduction not implicated in automatic response.

The Morphology and Physiology of the Telencephalon

The telencephalon is blanketed by the gray matter of the neocortex. This gray-colored concentration of nerve cells, which comprises the thin neocortical sheet, exhibits a high degree of morphological uniformity throughout its considerable expanse. The nerve cells of the neocortex are organized in a succession of six layers that display four distinct types of cellular architecture and three discernible tracts of axonal fibers (see Figure 11).

The surface of the cortex consists of a layer of axonal fibers covering the dense molecular layer of cortical neurons. Below the molecular layer of neurons are the layers of small and large pyramidal nerve cells, in that vertical sequence, distinguishable from one another through cell body size. The second band of axonal fibers projects through the layer of large pyramidal cells, whereas the third of the distinctive axonal tracts separates these large pyramidal cells from the deepest level of cortical nerve cell, the polymorphous layer. The neocortex exhibits extensive vertical and horizontal integration both through the transverse and vertical orientation of the three bands of axonal fibers, which are both myelinated and unmyelinated, and through the horizontal and vertical ramifications of the dendritic and axonal processes of the nerve cells within each layer of neocortex.

Two main types of association fibers, in addition to the transverse integration exhibited within the cortical gray matter, greatly enhance horizontal conduction within each cerebral hemisphere. Located directly

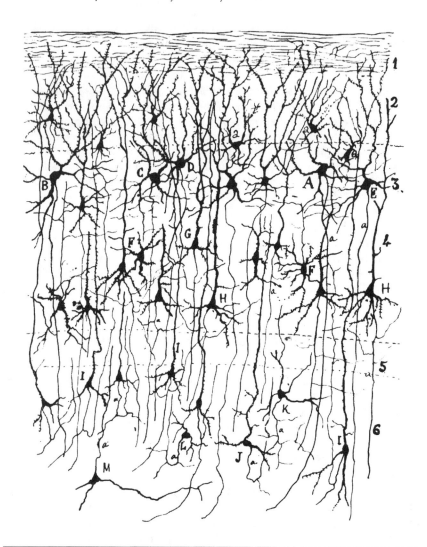

Figure 11. A sketch by Cajal (1888) of golgi-stained nerve tissue from the visual cortex of a rat. The numbers along the right margin refer to the six major cellular layers of the cortex, and the capital letters label individual cortical neurons. The human cortex also reflects these six cellular layers. From ''The Brain'' (p. 50) by David Hubel. Copyright © 1979 by Scientific American, Inc. All rights reserved.

beneath the polymorphous layer of neocortical neurons are the short association fibers, which project between adjacent convolutions of the cortex. In addition, long association fibers exist at even deeper levels within the cerebrum, directly connecting remote cortical areas. Paramount among these long association tracts are the following projections: the uncinate fasciculus, connecting the frontal lobe and the anterior temporal lobe; the superior longitudinal fasciculus, connecting the frontal and occipital and the frontal and temporal lobes; the inferior longitudinal fasciculus, connecting the temporal and occipital lobes; the perpendicular fasciculus, connecting the parietal and temporal lobes; the cingulum, connecting the hippocampal convolution and the callosal convolution; and the fornix, connecting the hippocampal convolution and deeper diencephalic centers. Both the fornix and the cingulum appear insinuated at points into the corpus callosum, suggesting further lateral, hemispherical integration in the conjunction of these association tracts.

Three aspects of cortical integration bear emphasis. First, horizontal and vertical integration within each convolution appears to be accomplished through the transverse and vertical dendritic and axonal processes invaginated within the cortical gray matter. Recent experimentation on the visual cortex of monkeys suggests that, for a particular episode of conduction, vertical integration of the layers of neocortex is prevalent, whereas horizontal integration appears localized to a diameter of a few millimeters. Second, the short association tracts immediately underlying the cortical gray matter effectively integrate adjacent convolutions and provide a second conduction framework for the sequential transmission of neuronal impulses across the neocortical sheet. Third, the long association tracts provide direct connections between distant areas of the cortex. It is interesting to note that the major pathways of the long association fibers connect remote neocortical areas with the temporal lobes of the telencephalon, which are contiguous with the hippocampal convolutions and amygdalas. Not only, then, is the hippocampus "a destination for sequential projections that span the neocortical sheet" (Nauta & Feirtag, 1979, p. 52), but it also is located proximately to long association tracts connecting the temporal lobes with the frontal, occipital, and parietal lobes. And the hippocampus, in turn, appears well integrated with the important diencephalic processing centers through major parallel projection tracts, such as the fornix and cingulum.

The two quasisymmetrical hemispheres of the telencephalon are separated by the longitudinal fissure. The tracts that traverse this fissure, comprised mostly of myelinated axons, are called commissures, of which the corpus callosum is by far the largest and most important. The corpus callosum contains parallel fibers that conduct impulses in both transverse directions. These fibers of the corpus callosum radiate throughout each hemisphere, presumably connecting each peripheral region of neocortex with the corresponding region within the opposing hemisphere. Hemispherical integration also is accomplished through lesser commissures, of which the anterior commissure is the most notable. The anterior commissure consists of a bundle of myelinated axonal fibers that appear to connect, through reciprocal projections, the corpus striatum of one hemisphere with that same region of the opposing hemisphere. The two hemispheres of the temporal lobes of the telencephalon therefore appear to be bridged most proximately by the anterior commissure. The axonal processes of the cortex, in other words, are oriented primarily in three directions. Bridging the otherwise complete division between the cerebral hemispheres are the connecting tracts called commissures. Horizontal, or transverse, neuronal integration within the telencephalon involves conduction primarily along association tracts, which are bundles of myelinated axons of varying lengths. Finally, the thalamic centers within the diencephalon radiate myelinated axons to and from all cortical areas. These projection tracts are called the corona radiata, and they provide direct vertical integration between the gray matter of the cortex and the diencephalic processing centers.

Cerebral integration, in addition to neuronal integration along these many major nerve tracts, is presumed to involve substantial axonal and dendritic conduction between the smaller and frequently unmyelinated neurons of the neocortex and the many other deeper nerve cell centers. Some recent speculation also suggests the possibility that neuronal conduction pathways may include nonneuronal mediums such as the glial cells and the ventricular spaces within the brain. Indeed Penfield (1975) suggested the possibility of nonneuronal conduction some years ago: "One may ask the question: does the highest brain mechanism provide the mind with its energy, an energy in such a changed form that it no longer needs to be conducted along neuraxones?" (p. 56).

The physiology of the telencephalon is poorly understood. Functions appear to be localized to particular geographical areas of the neocortex but only in a rather general and peculiar way. The physiological mapping of the neocortex has occupied neurophysiologists for over a century, however, and a substantial body of information has been compiled.

The most obvious anatomical division within the telencephalon is its separation by the longitudinal fissure into the two relatively symmetrical cerebral hemispheres. Much recent research has focused on the lateralization of functions between the two hemispheres.

It has long been recognized that the primary afferent and efferent nerve tracts cross before entering and after leaving the brain. These peripheral nerve tracts exhibit a bilateral symmetry along the axis of the spine, and, with few exceptions, the crossing of the nerve pathways effectively links the left side of the body to the right cerebral hemisphere and the right side of the body to the left cerebral hemisphere. The discoveries by Paul Broca and Carl Wernicke that the mechanisms for speech tend to localize in the left cerebral hemisphere, especially in right-handed individuals, marked the first real recognition that hemispherical specialization might be more than a mirror image of the bilateral symmetry of the peripheral nervous system.

The information relating to hemispherical specialization comes from analysis of individuals who have sustained either extensive damage or disease process to one hemisphere only or from experimentation with individuals who have had the principal nerve tract connecting the hemispheres, the corpus callosum, surgically severed by a commissurotomy, a last-resort method of controlling grand mal epilepsy. Although the analytical data are far from conclusive, several strong indications of specialized hemispheric function have emerged.

For the vast majority of the population, the left hemisphere demonstrates an analytical, logical cognitive framework, whereas the right hemisphere applies a holistic, Gestalt framework of cognition. The fundamental cognitive difference can be understood to involve the left hemisphere's specialization in a system of temporal conceptual processing, as distinguished from the right hemisphere's specialization in spatial conceptualization. Spatial processing defines the limits and orientation of an object within the three dimensions of space. Temporal processing defines the changes in the spatial limits and orientation of an object over time and introduces the concept of causation that underpins all analytical and logical processes and that is itself grounded in memory. Such hemispheric specialization is by no means absolute, however, for the evidence suggests that each hemisphere contains the capacity for conceptualization involving both time and space. In fact, "split-brain" research has demonstrated that each of the hemispheres in a commissurotomized subject will perceive, learn, and respond independently of the other hemisphere. The separated hemispheres even seem to embody independent and occasionally antagonistic states of consciousness.

In the normal individual, of course, the two hemispheres are integrated by the several hemispherical commissures, especially the corpus callosum. Presumably, such lateral integration permits the specialized frameworks of conceptualization localized to each hemisphere to operate synergistically such that greater resolution is achieved in placing the conceptual object in both time and space.

Just as the cerebrum is divided hemispherically, the anterior and posterior parts of the cortex are separated by a deep fissure called the central sulcus. Immediately anterior to the central sulcus is the area localized from birth for motor response, called the precentral gyrus. Immediately posterior to the central sulcus is the area localized from birth for somatic sensory reception, called the postcentral gyrus. These two areas are the motor cortex and the somatosensory cortex, respectively, and they both have been mapped to a high degree of resolution. In general, the maps of the somatosensory and the motor cortices mirror each other across the central sulcus.

Figure 12 illustrates the areas of specialization discovered within the somatic sensory and motor regions of the cerebral cortex. Discrete functional parts of the body are associated with specific areas of the somatic sensory and motor regions, as reflected in the distorted homunculi depicted. The distortions schematically illustrate that the extent of the cortical area dedicated to a particular part of the body is proportional to the precision of control required rather than to the size of the part. Only one half of each cortical area is shown, as the missing halves are virtual mirror images of the halves depicted (and are associated with the opposite side of the body).

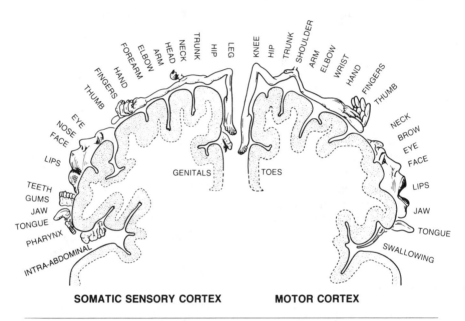

SOMATIC SENSORY CORTEX   **MOTOR CORTEX**

Figure 12.   A diagram illustrating specialization within the somatic sensory and motor regions of the cerebral cortex. *Note.* From "Specialization of the Human Brain" (p. 182) by N. Geschwind. Copyright © 1979 by Scientific American, Inc. All rights reserved.

Within the anterior cerebrum, which consists principally of the frontal lobe, most functions appear to relate to motor response, including the formation of intent, intellectual or abstract reasoning, and language and speech. Areas of the posterior cerebrum, on the other hand, appear to be related more directly to sensory perception and integration. The parietal lobes, which include the somatosensory cortex of the postcentral gyrus together with the temporal lobes, appear to relate present sensory experience to past sensory experiences stored in memory. The cortical area that functions as a primary processing center for the sense of taste is located near the lowest point of the postcentral gyrus, whereas the primary cortical processing stations for hearing and olfaction are localized within the temporal lobes. The cortical center for the sense of vision is located in the most posterior area of the telencephalon within the occipital lobes. Memory appears to be distributed throughout the cortex.

Centrencephalic Integration

What emerges from a review of the current information with respect to brain physiology is an appreciation of the extraordinary integration of the various brain areas in the performance of conceptually discrete functions. Penfield has termed this pervasive system of functional association "centrencephalic integration":

> *I have referred to the system of connections that must serve the integrative activity that comes between the sensory input, into the diencephalon, and the motor output as the centrencephalic system. Within that integrating system there is an automatic computer and a mechanism that makes consciousness possible. When the specialized areas of the cerebral cortex are in action, some of them at least are as much involved in the neurone action related to consciousness as is the diencephalon.* (Penfield, 1975, p. 56)

Penfield suggests, in other words, that both automatic and conscious brain functions, ranging from sensory perception to motor response, are best understood as the product of patterns of centrencephalic integration.

The Physiology of Sensory Perception

Sensory perception in humans is presumed to involve multiple levels of neural processing. The mechanisms of perception vary between the different sensoria. In addition, sensory impulses originating in the same sensory receptors can vary substantially between separate episodes of stimulation. Consequently, neurophysiologists are only beginning to discern the complex patterns of centrencephalic integration involved in sensory perception. It is abundantly clear, however, that most acts of sensory perception cannot be localized to unitary, anatomically distinct areas of the brain.

Recent experimentation involving the processes of visual perception in monkeys suggests that the visual cortex contains localized processing centers specific to a particular aspect of visual perception. So, for example, certain delimited columnar organizations of neocortical neurons appear to be activated in response to a precise stimulus within the visual field, such as the spatial orientation or direction of movement of a line segment. Such experimental findings have led theorists to conclude that the sensory cortex has localized, specific "feature detectors," which respond to specific sensory stimuli. The association and interpretation of these features into an act of sensory perception, however, is understood to involve far more extensive processes of centrencephalic integration.

Afferent impulses from most sensoria are first processed through centers within both the reticular formation and the thalamus before being projected to the telencephalon. Sensory input to the thalamus potentially is projected through the reciprocated thalamocortical tract to the appropriate sensory cortex of the telencephalon. In addition, the corona radiata provides parallel projection tracts directly integrating the thalamic centers with multiple remote neocortical regions. Horizontal integration of the various cortical areas entrained by projections from the thalamus potentially involves both conduction along the reciprocated long and short association tracts that run in the cerebral white matter beneath the neocortical sheet and a "neocortical march" involving sequential conduction within the gray matter of the neocortical sheet itself.

Experimentation involving the implantation of electrodes within the various brain centers of monkeys in order to record temporal and spatial patterns of electrical discharge in response to visual stimuli suggests that visual perception involves a convergent process of centrencephalic integration. Visual images are coded for transmission to the brain within an ordered variety of retinal cells linked in a sophisticated synaptic network. The optic nerves project from these ganglion cells of the retina directly (subject only to reordering through a partial crossover at the optic chiasm) to the lateral geniculate nuclei of the thalamus. From this cellular interrupt in the lateral geniculate nucleus, transmissions are projected without interruption to the visual cortex in the posterior occipital lobe. The processing of visual input transmission within the visual cortex becomes extremely complex but appears to involve a sequence of localized feature detectors. From the visual cortex, transmissions are projected to adjacent and remote regions of the neocortex and to centers deep within the brain. Prominent among these latter projections are nerve tracts that return, or feed back, to the lateral geniculate nucleus. Several commentators have suggested, on the basis of these experiments involving microelectrode implantation, that visual perception involves a convergence and integration of sensory input from the retinal ganglion cells with memory-based interpretive feedback generated within various cortical areas (most notably, the visual cortex, the posterior association cortex, and the inferior temporal cortex).

Pribram has hypothesized an integrative process modeled on the optical phenomenon of holography, in which perception is understood to be a function of the interference patterns generated by the superposition of electrochemical waves representing sensory input and interpretive feedback (Pribram, 1981, p. 108). Pribram's holographic model views the processes of perception from a holistic, macrosystemic perspective. Although interesting and provocative, the holographic model is extremely abstract and inchoate. Pribram also has analyzed perception on the cellular and molecular microsystemic levels, however, and this analysis has yielded a far more definite conception of the integral mechanism of perception. Pribram's model of sensory perception posits neuronal microsystems termed "feature analyzers," which coordinate and integrate the hard-wired "feature detectors" that correspond to such basic physical properties as color, contour, movement, and spatial orientation. The feature analyzers are conceived as "memory units" that associate, integrate, and interpret neuronal information processed through the built-in feature detectors. The feature detectors are believed by Pribram to be columnar organizations of cortical neurons that respond to a specific receptive field, giving rise to a particular neuronal coding, or "unit of representation of the input," from the receptive field. The process by which these columnar units of representation are integrated and interpreted Pribram models as TOTE servomechanisms. A TOTE servomechanism (i.e., Test-Operate-Test-Exit) is a cybernetic system, such as a thermostat, that permits feedforward information and feedback information to be equilibrated. Pribram suggests that TOTE servomechanisms constitute the basic unit (or microsystem) or neurobehavioral analysis:

> A generalized diagram of the reflex, the unit of neurobehavioral analysis, can therefore be attempted. . . . To be effective, input must be compared to and tested against spontaneous or corollary central neural activity; the results of this comparison initiate some operation which then influences either other parts of the nervous system or the external world. The consequences of this operation are then fed back to the comparator and the loop continues until the test has been satisfied—until some previous setting, indicative of a state-to-be-achieved, has been attained (exit). . . . The Test phase of the logic expresses the junctional, the Operate phase the nerve-impulse portion of the two-process mechanism of brain function. (Pribram, 1981, pp. 93-96)

Pribram hypothesizes that the integration of the various feature detectors is accomplished through the equilibration of feedforward and feedback information within neuronal TOTE servomechanisms, or feature analyzers. The "Test" phase of the feature analysis process is a function of the state of the junctional microstructure, or synapse. That state, in turn, is determined both by the evolved structure and conformation of the synapse and by the electrochemical milieu generated by the perfusion of neurotransmitters into that synapse. This "slow potential junctional microstructure," as Pribram terms it, constitutes the "bias" of the Test phase. The bias therefore can be influenced by the action of remote regions of the brain that cause either excitatory or inhibitory neurotransmitters to enter the synapse of the feature analyzer.

The conception of sensory perception that Pribram develops, therefore, involves intricate, localized systems of feature analysis that are tuned and modulated by the action of remote cortical regions. The temporal cortex and amygdaloid complex, for example, are understood to enhance the neural mechanisms involved in lateral inhibition between the "logic elements" of the remote feature analyzers. They achieve this effect by virtue of the specific inhibitory or excitatory effect of the neurotransmitter that is released into the synapses of the feature analysis mechanisms from the presynaptic terminals of their axonal projections. In other words, a particular junctional microstructure involved in an episode of sensory perception may appear relatively local, yet neuraxones that synapse within and thereby affect that junctional microstructure potentially originate in remote brain centers. Moreover, with the recent discovery that many neurotransmitters also function as hormones, the possibility arises that transport of neurotransmitters/hormones through the bloodstream and the cerebrospinal fluid may provide an additional mechanism for remote modulation of the synapses within the feature analysis microsystems. At any rate, this conception of the mechanisms involved in sensory perception suggests an extremely complex and potentially pervasive system of centrencephalic integration. Even the apparently local microsystems hypothesized to operate as feature detectors and analyzers appear to be influenced substantially from remote neural centers.

Physicist and neurophysiologist Erich Harth offers a similar but less abstract model to explain the mechanism of convergent processing. Harth analyzes the physiology of visual perception to illustrate the integration of sensory input and interpretive feedback that he believes to be common to virtually all sensory perception. In general, Harth's model identifies certain focal areas within the brain that synthesize or equilibrate neuronal information received from the sensoria and from memory. Specifically, Harth cites Wolf Singer's characterization of the lateral geniculate nucleus as an "inner retina," which reflects a distribution of neuronal activity over its constituent sheets of neurons that substantially replicates the patterns of neuronal activity within the retina. Harth points out that the corticofugal fibers that project to the lateral geniculate nucleus from the retina are extremely similar in number and spatial distribution to the parallel fibers that run between the lateral geniculate nucleus and the visual cortex. Moreover, "there is evidence that the returning messages [from the cortex] are feature specific; that is, they can enhance, select, and perhaps mimic sensory patterns." Harth suggests, principally on the basis of these observations, that the lateral geniculate nucleus, which he abbreviates as LGN, functions as an "internal sketchpad": "The idea is that sensory patterns are laid down in the LGN by sensory input, but similar patterns may also be sketched there by higher centers. The LGN is a possible location for such a process, but certainly not the only place where this may occur'' (Harth, 1982, pp. 172-173). The lateral geniculate nucleus therefore is posited as a location for the integration of sensory input and interpretive feedback. Harth hypothesizes an integrative mechanism of feature enhancement called a "neural Alopex process" (Harth, 1982, pp. 174-177). Similar processes of integration and equilibration are posited as the mechanisms of all sensory perception.

The descriptions of the precise mechanisms for the synthesis and integration of sensory input and memory, such as Pribram's feature analyzers and holographic superposition and Harth's neural Alopex process, are highly speculative. Yet, however it might work, some such mechanism of centrencephalic integration almost certainly underpins all complex sensory perception.

Conceptually, it is possible to distinguish between processes of sensory perception that proceed automatically without an attendant sense of awareness and those that are characterized by conscious awareness in the form of attention. The physiological basis for such a distinction, although by no means obvious or well settled, can be extrapolated from an analysis of the various neural pathways involved in sensory perception.

It can be hypothesized that processes of perception that implicate only the relatively delimited neural circuitry of the thalamus and the appropriate sensory cortex and that can be presumed to interface with proximate effector systems within the motor cortex—either directly or through the thalamic centers—proceed automatically, without an accompanying subjective sense of attention. The vast preponderance of sensory perception is of this nature, proceeding without conscious awareness.

Alternatively, those processes of perception that involve widespread horizontal integration of diffuse associative and interpretive areas of the neocortex and that generally include integration with the subcortical areas of the hippocampus and amygdala can be hypothesized to induce an accompanying sense of conscious awareness, manifest as attention. The subjective sensation of attention, therefore, is conceived as a phenomenon attendant upon the transcortical processes underlying sensory perception.

Recent experimentation in computer-averaged electroencephalography (EEG) provides some support for this supposition. Electroencephalography, until the advent of computer-averaging techniques, was far too crude a measurement device to permit the discernment of generalized electrical brain responses to specific stimuli. A particular stimulus-response pattern would be lost to detection and measurement in the background "noise" of general brain activity. Through EEG-monitored repetition of a specific stimulus-response pattern over time, however, a body of information could be generated from which computer-assisted analysis could extract the average response pattern from the average background noise. Researchers employing such computer-averaged EEG techniques discovered a dramatic increase in generalized neocortical electrical activity when the experimental subject was actively attempting but unable to extract a conceptual pattern from a sensory stimulus. They termed this widespread cortical excitation an "evoked potential." The evoked potential can be interpreted as a transcortical manifestation of the neural processes underlying sensory perception. Such extensive centrencephalic integration appears necessarily partnered with an accompanying subjective sense of awareness in the form of attention (Restak, 1979, pp. 283-289).

Additional experimental support for the proposition that conscious perception requires sustained and widespread cortical activity comes from experiments by neurophysiologist Benjamin Libet. Libet used computer-averaged EEG techniques to measure the evoked potential related to conscious perception of a sensory stimulus. Libet concluded, among other things, that "conscious response to a stimulus cannot occur . . . unless some form of neuronal reverberation continues for up to about half a second, the 'adequate' time for sensation" (Harth, 1982, pp. 201-202). This distinction between complex sensory perception that is not accompanied by attentive awareness and complex sensory perception that is attended by subjective awareness will be explored at greater length later in this chapter.

The Physiology of Motor Response

Centrencephalic integration is nowhere more apparent than in the process of human motor response. Again, however, it appears possible to distinguish between motor responses that are automatic and those that are volitional, and the functional distinction can be presumed to turn on the extent of neocortical involvement in the processes of centrencephalic integration.

The vast preponderance of motor response is, of course, automatic, occurring outside the focus of awareness. Experimentation upon monkeys has suggested that a repertoire of discrete muscular responses is stored somehow within the lower-brain centers, spinal cord, and peripheral neural processes. Bilateral surgical removal of even the entire motor cortex in monkeys does not preclude all motor response. In fact, the integrity of specific, constituent muscular movements appears relatively unimpaired, despite bilateral extirpation of the motor cortex. However, the capacity for coordination of such basic integral movements into more complex, task-oriented contractile patterns appears to be eliminated entirely.

Anatomical and physiological evidence suggests a similar organization of the motor system in humans. It is presumed that a repertoire of basic, integral motor responses is stored within the neural centers of the lower brain, spinal cord, and peripheral neural processes. Nauta and Feirtag have conceptualized the peripheral, or lower, motor system as comprised of what they term "local motor apparatuses": "Each local motor apparatus is, it seems, a kind of file room in which blueprints, each one representing a possible movement of a particular body part, are stored. The brain, with its descending fiber systems, reaches down and selects the appropriate blueprint" (Nauta & Feirtag, 1979, p. 50).

The local motor apparatuses appear to be discrete functional systems organized in the form of biasable reflex processes. In other words, the reflex loops that innervate a particular local motor apparatus are not functionally autonomous. Instead, they almost always are susceptible to modulation through cybernetic feedback systems operating both peripherally and centrally.

The archetypical example of a reflex system is the "closed-loop," or "monosynaptic reflex arc," in which a primary sensory neuron directly excites a motor neuron. Such monosynaptic reflexes are found in phylogenetically primitive organisms as well as in certain peripheral proprioceptive systems in humans. Obviously, the reflex arcs that comprise the human repertoire of local motor apparatuses cannot operate strictly as closed-loop systems. Such an organization of the neural motor system would preclude any central coordination of movement. Yet the available evidence demonstrates that the brain's orchestration of coordinated motor response is almost always accomplished through a neural exchange that occurs on the sensory side of the reflex arc rather than through direct neural control over the arc's motor neuron. The reflex arc, therefore, remains substantially intact, but supraspinal modulations of the sensitivity or bias of the sensory neuron within that arc effectively control the excitation of the motor neuron. Such a system of centralized control of the repertoire of local motor apparatuses is entirely dependent on an active exchange of neural information between the sensory neuron of the reflex arc—that is, the proprioceptor mechanism—and the brain centers that modulate the sensitivity of that sensory neuron. This system of centralized cybernetic control operates through the sensory feedback transmitted from the sensory neuron in its proprioceptor mode. In fact, the contractile process within a muscle is only rarely initiated by direct supraspinal excitation of the contractile fibers. Instead, neural control of muscular contraction is affected in most instances through modulations in the biases of the cybernetic microsystems that comprise a muscle's proprioceptor system.

The principal proprioceptor mechanisms involved in this contractile process appear to be the muscle spindles, which are integrated into a cybernetic system through the gamma efferent neural system. A muscle spindle consists of a small number (3 to 10) of muscle fibers, called intrafusal fibers, together with two types of stretch receptors, all encapsulated in a membranous sheath and interspersed within the contractile, or extrafusal, fibers of a muscle. These highly specialized sensory organs are designed to respond to any stretching of the muscle in which they are embedded by stimulating a reflexive contraction of that muscle. The contractile mechanisms within the intrafusal fibers are located at the polar ends of the spindle, whereas the stretch receptors occupy the central region of the spindle. Each spindle possesses two distinct types of receptor mechanisms, one of which monitors spindle length and the other the rate of change in spindle length. Because muscle length varies over such a large range, the spindles must adjust, or equilibrate, to any particular muscle length in order to register a variation from that length. The gamma efferent neural system stimulates the intrafusal fibers to contract in response to shortenings of muscle length, thereby keeping the muscle spindle length tuned to the muscle length in such a way that its proprioceptor function remains operant. The degree to which the length of the intrafusal fibers are modulated by the gamma efferent system constitutes the bias of the system.

The most common method of neural control over muscular contraction involves modulation of the bias on the intrafusal fibers rather than direct excitation of the extrafusal fibers. In other words, the contraction of the polar ends of the intrafusal fibers in response to supraspinal stimulation through the gamma efferent system will activate the stretch receptor mechanism within the central region of the spindle, triggering a reflexive contraction of the extrafusal muscle fibers.

Figure 13 is a schematic diagram of the gamma efferent contractile system. The "bias" of this cybernetic system is controlled through input from the higher centers to the gamma motor neuron (1), causing a shortening of the polar ends of the intrafusal fibers (2), thereby activating the stretch receptor mechanism within the central region of the spindle (3), which then excites the alpha motor neuron (4), ultimately causing contraction of the extrafusal fiber (5).

The integral unit for most muscular contraction, then, is understood to be the cybernetic microsystem involving the muscle spindles and the reflex loop to the extrafusal muscle fibers. And, of course, the coordination of the numerous cybernetic microsystems throughout the body is achieved through processes of centrencephalic integration within the brain.

As in the preceding analysis of sensory perception, it is possible to hypothesize a physiological foundation for distinguishing complex motor activity not attended by awareness from complex motor activity accompanied by awareness.

The automatic sensory-motor mechanism identified by Penfield appears to involve neural circuitry that engages a selection of local motor appa-

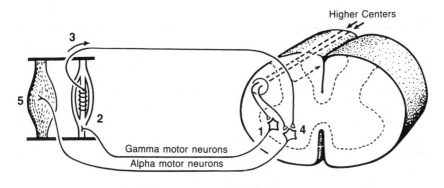

Figure 13. A schematic diagram of the gamma efferent contractile system. *Note.* Reprinted by permission of the publisher from *Principles of Neural Science* (p. 299), edited by E.R. Kandel and J.W. Swartz. Copyright 1985 by Elsevier Science Publishing Co., Inc.

ratuses through projections originating within a process of centrencephalic integration that includes the motor and the sensory cortices, the corpus striatum, and the cerebellum and that is mediated through the thalamus. The involvement of the corpus striatum and cerebellum in coordinated motor response originally was suggested by pathological evidence correlating damage to either structure with severe and distinctive impairments of motor coordination. More recently, experiments involving the implantation of microelectrodes within the corpus striata and cerebella of monkeys have demonstrated that these areas are electrically active immediately prior to coordinated motor response. Through the mechanisms of such an integrated circuitry—monitored through proprioceptive feedback to the somatosensory and the motor cortices, the cerebellum, and the corpus striatum—highly skilled and precise movements can be achieved without an attendant sense of conscious awareness. In fact, once a complex motor skill has been learned, it generally can be performed more proficiently without the involvement of subjective awareness.

Volitional motor response, on the other hand, appears to implicate a far more extensive involvement of the neocortex in the system of centrencephalic integration. As indicated above, virtually the entire neocortex projects uninterrupted neural tracts to both the corpus striatum (often referred to as the basal ganglia) and the pons. The corpus striatum subjects these cortical inputs to several layers of internal processing involving the striatum and the globus pallidus before projecting a major branch of the ansa lenticularis in a semicircular loop to the anterior portion of the thalamus. The pons projects a massive neural tract to the cerebellum, which in turn projects to the thalamus by the way of the brachium conjunctivum. These inputs are projected to the premotor and the motor cortices from the thalamus. After cortical processing in the precentral motor gyrus, volitional motor signals are projected to the effector neurons of the appropriate selection of local motor apparatuses either directly through the corticospinal tract or by way of the reticular formation. And as in automatic functions, proprioceptive sensory systems are believed to provide cybernetic feedback not only to the motor and somatosensory cortex but also to both the corpus striatum and the cerebellum.

The distinction between volitional and automatic motor response is not easily made. Nauta and Feirtag, for example, suggest that "the motor system almost defies examination from the standpoint of volitional behavior, as opposed to nonvolitional" (Nauta & Feirtag, 1979, p. 51). Edward Evarts, on the other hand, in pursuing that examination, declares his agreement with the view of Swedish neurophysiologist Ragnar Granit that "what is volitional in voluntary movement is its purpose." Evarts hypothesizes that the achievement of any such purpose is, however, "built up from a variety of reflex processes" (Evarts, 1979, p. 106).

An understanding of volitional motor response consequently is most productively pursued through an investigation of the subjective sense of purpose that most clearly distinguishes volitional response from automatic response. It has long been observed that extensive damage to the frontal lobes of the cerebrum—through injury, disease, or surgical intrusion—causes a loss of a subjective sense of purpose in the individual. Research has confirmed that goal-directed intention and volition are integrally related to the proper functioning of the frontal cortex. These functions, however, appear to be dispersed over wide cortical areas and are certainly not precisely localized. For example, Penfield's extensive electrical mapping experiments demonstrated that "there is no place in the cerebral cortex where electrical stimulation will cause a patient to believe or to decide" (Penfield, 1975, p. 77).

These observations have been confirmed and refined by recent experimentation by H. H. Kornhuber and his colleagues involving the electrical mapping of neuronal activity immediately preceding a voluntary motor response (specifically, the voluntary flexion of a forefinger). This revealing work has demonstrated the existence of a bilateral electrical potential throughout the cerebral cortex that seems to correspond to the formulation of intent or volition. This electrical potential, called the "readiness potential," arises approximately .8 seconds before voluntary muscle action, displays a gradual increase in intensity, and involves widespread neuronal activity throughout both cerebral hemispheres. Yet another positive potential, called the "premotion positive potential," arises bilaterally about 90 milliseconds before muscle action. Approximately 50 milliseconds before muscle action, an electrical potential indicating neuronal activity is detected that is localized to the area of the motor cortex corresponding to the muscle groups to be activated (Harth, 1982, 165-169; Restak, 1979, pp. 243-244).

The process of volitional muscle response can be hypothesized on the basis of this experimental evidence to include three distinct stages. First, the readiness potential appears to correspond to the abstracted process of construction of intent or volition. The frontal and temporal lobes can be presumed to be integral to this process of intent formulation though by no means an exclusive locus for it. Second, the premotion positive potential can be understood to represent neuronal integration between the diffuse neocortical regions involved in the readiness potential and those brain areas directly involved in coordinated motor functions: the cerebellum, the corpus striatum, and the motor and the somatosensory cortices. The premotion positive potential therefore can be conceived to involve the codification of intent into an integrated program for motor response. Such a process of centrencephalic integration presumably would be mediated through the diencephalon. Finally, just before muscle activity is manifest, the integrated program is reflected in a pattern of neuronal activity in the appropriate area of the motor cortex.

Harth has suggested a slightly different interpretation of the Kornhuber experiments. Harth hypothesizes that the nearly 1 second of discernible electrical activity preceding voluntary motor response involves the formulation of what he terms a proprioceptive schema:

> *What, then, goes on in the brain during that relatively long stretch of one second preceding this spontaneous voluntary action? We cannot be sure, but we will make a guess. The flexing of the forefinger, like any action, is accompanied by a variety of sensory responses, visual and skin responses, plus the internal senses of muscle, joint, and tendon. Together they constitute a sensory pattern, a schema. . . . Let us call it a proprioceptive schema.* (Harth, 1979, p. 168)

In other words, Harth views the readiness and premotion potentials as electrochemical processes that compile and coordinate the proprioceptive schema for an intended motor act. Harth identifies the somatosensory cortex as the primary location in which the proprioceptive schema is patterned, suggesting that "the spillover of the growing somatosensory activity across the central sulcus into the motor region will eventually precipitate the action itself" (Harth, 1982, p. 168).

Pribram also has expounded a theory of volitional motor activity. Complex movements are presumed by Pribram to be coordinated through mechanisms within the motor cortex that exert central control over the tonal bias state orchestrated through the basal ganglia and cerebellum. Experimentation has demonstrated that the neural connections between the peripheral servomechanisms and these brain centers are coded in terms of force relationships: "Because reflexes are constituted of servomechanisms, their central representations are constructed not of records of muscle length or tension, but of the parameters of adjustment and compensation to the changing external forces involved in the activity" (Pribam, 1981, p. 248). Pribram hypothesizes that the anterior cerebellum, because of its unique cellular architecture, functions as a fast-time comparator to compute an approximate projection of past and current force relationships into future consequences—that is, to compute "a rough sketching out of the operations to be performed" (Pribram, 1981, p. 232). The anterior cerebellum, therefore, is understood to compute "the end point of a convergent series" that is coded in terms of force relationships and fed forward to the motor cortex, where it arises in consciousness as an "Image-of-Achievement." The Image-of-Achievement, then, is conceived to program the biases of peripheral servomechanisms in order to produce voluntary or volitional motor activity. Pribram offers the following synopsis of his model of volitional behavior:

> A momentary Image-of-Achievement is constructed and continuously updated through a neural holographic process much as is the perceptual Image. The Image-of-Achievement is, however, composed of learned anticipations of the force and changes in force required to perform a task. These fields of force exerted on muscle receptors become the parameters of the servomechanisms and are directly (via the thalamus) and indirectly (via the basal ganglia and cerebellum) relayed to the motor cortex, where they are correlated with a fast-time cerebellar computation to predict the outcomes of the next steps of the action. When the course of action becomes reasonably predictable from the trends of prior successful predictions, a terminal Image-of-Achievement can be constituted to serve as a guide for the final phases of the activity. (Pribram, 1981, pp. 249-250)

All of the preceding hypotheses concerning the processes of centrencephalic integration involved in volitional motor response are highly speculative. Yet a modest retreat to firmer theoretical ground still suggests that volitional movement implicates a far greater range and duration of neocortical activity than does automatic motor response. Although the subjective experience of volition appears intimately related to extensive neocortical activity, especially involving the frontal and temporal lobes, automatic motor activity seems substantially limited to the motor and sensory neocortical areas.

The Physiology of Memory

The subjective sense of purpose or volition is a fundamental manifestation of conscious awareness. Yet a necessary precondition for any subjective experience that might meaningfully be characterized as awareness, including volition, is that specialized process of mind called memory.

As with other functions associated with operations of mind, the physiology of memory is not well understood. Most current speculation presumes that memory involves morphological changes that affect principally the synaptic and ephaptic junctions between neurons. It is hypothesized that the passage of a neuronal impulse activates, frequently by means of a second-messenger mechanism, certain molecular adaptations within either the presynaptic or the postsynaptic terminals. These transformational processes, which are believed to be mediated by RNA, reorder cellular protein configurations in ways that are functionally significant to the junctional interface between neurons. In particular, such adaptations are believed to modify the synaptic processes by altering the conformation of the synaptic gating mechanisms involved in the presynaptic release and postsynaptic reception of neurotransmitter and by altering the rate of synthesis or decomposition of neurotransmitter. Additionally, memory formation is understood to involve an increase in the glial cells surrounding the nerve cells, and it is hypothesized that this discernible proliferation of glial cells facilitates axonal conduction within the enveloped neurons.

It is natural to assume that the processes of memory that underpin the human experience of conscious awareness are qualitatively different from the processes of memory on which the conditioned learning responses of the phylogenetically lower animals are based. Experimentation and analysis has revealed, however, that such a distinction may be unwarranted. Not only do "there appear to be no fundamental differences in structure, chemistry or function between the neurons and synapses in man and those of a squid, a snail or a leech" (Kandel, 1979, p. 29), but recent investigations suggest that neural mechanisms of learning may be functionally equivalent as well.

Much of the research concerning the physiology of learning has focused on animals that possess relatively simple nervous systems that are experimentally accessible and manageable. Neurophysiologist Eric Kandel and his colleagues have investigated the rote learning processes involved in habituation and sensitization within the limited neural systems of the large marine snail *Aplysia*. Their findings are extremely provocative.

Habituation consists of a progressive decrease in the magnitude of an organism's behavioral response as the number of repetitions of a particular stimulus increases. When the stimulus is innocuous, with neither favorable nor unfavorable implications for the organism's well-being or survival, habituation to the stimulus can be characterized as learning.

Kandel and his colleagues studied habituation processes involving the monosynaptic reflex response of gill withdrawal in *Aplysia*. Habituation, they determined, is caused by a progressive decrease in the neurotransmitter released from the presynaptic sensory neuron. This measurable decrease in the release of neurotransmitter corresponds to a detectable decrease in the calcium ion current generated by an action potential within the presynaptic terminal. Apparently, repeated stimulation of the sensory neuron sufficient to cause habituation produces a decreasing calcium current within the presynaptic terminal and a consequent decrease in transmitter release into the synaptic gap. The connection between the sensory neuron and the motor neuron that constitutes the monosynaptic reflex arc is therefore progressively disrupted through processes of habituation. Kandel found no qualitative basis for distinguishing between short- and long-term habituation. Instead, habituation of longer duration appeared to be a result of greater frequency and more episodes of the habituating stimulus but to involve the same neuronal mechanisms as the more transient patterns of habituation.

Sensitization is the learning process directly opposed to habituation. It consists of a progressive enhancement of an organism's behavioral response as the number of repetitions of a particular stimulus increases. When the stimulus carries either favorable or unfavorable implications for the organism's well-being and survival, an appropriate sensitization to the stimulus can be characterized as learning.

Kandel and his associates determined that the mechanisms of sensitization relating to gill withdrawal behavior in *Aplysia* also are localized in the presynaptic terminal but involve an entirely distinct process from habituation. Neurons external to the monosynaptic reflex arc synapse on the presynaptic terminal of the sensory neuron. These external neurons, which intervene in that reflex arc, are called interneurons. The interneurons were determined to modulate the sensitization process through their synaptic interface with the presynaptic terminal of the sensory neuron that triggers the motor neuron responsible for activating gill withdrawal.

The electrochemical processes involved in sensitization are more complex than those involved in habituation. Kandel has hypothesized a sensitization process that involves release of the neurotransmitter serotonin by the facilitating interneuron. The serotonin reacts with the presynaptic membrane of the sensory neuron to activate a membrane protein called adenylate cyclase, which in turn catalyzes the reduction of ATP within the presynaptic terminal of the sensory neuron to cyclic adenosine monophosphate (cyclic AMP). Cyclic AMP then acts as a "second messenger" to affect membrane-gating mechanisms that increase the calcium ion current into the presynaptic terminal of the sensory neuron, thereby increasing its release of neurotransmitter. The increased release of neurotransmitter facilitates the monosynaptic reflex arc, causing a sensitization of gill withdrawal behavior.

Both habituation and sensitization therefore can be understood to involve modulations in neurotransmitter release from presynaptic terminals. Changes involving membrane gating mechanisms— particularly those governing calcium ion current—appear to be the physiological bases for such modifications in synaptic conduction of neuronal impulses. Electron microscopy has revealed that habituation and sensitization within *Aplysia* frequently correlate with measurable structural adaptations within the neuronal microsystems involved in the stimulus-response reflex arc. Habituation and sensitization can be either short- or long-term, depending primarily on the magnitude and the frequency of the stimulus triggering the adaptive process.

It would be naive and presumptuous to conclude that all mechanisms of memory and learning conform precisely to these patterns. However, Kandel and his colleagues have demonstrated that elementary patterns of learning can be understood in the strictly mechanical terms of subcellular electrochemical processes. It is not unreasonable to assume that physiological processes like those governing the gill withdrawal reflex in *Aplysia* comprise what Kandel calls an "elementary alphabet of mentation" from which the language of all complex mental processes, including conscious awareness, might be derived (Kandel, 1979, p. 38).

Current theories concerning the encoding of memory are based on the considerable experimental evidence that memory formation correlates with discernible organic modifications within the brain. Specifically, it has been observed that memory formation corresponds to adaptations within the microsystemic linkages that form the conductive junctions between nerve cells and to the proliferation of the dendrite connections and glial cells surrounding the nerve cells. The available evidence indicates that memory formation does not involve an increase in the number of nerve cells and may even correspond in some instances to a selective elimination of nerve cells. In light of this evidence of a correlation between memory formation and modifications to the synaptic microsystems and the glial surround, it is hypothesized that memory is encoded by organic adaptations to physiological microsystems that affect both synaptic and axonal transmission of neuronal impulses.

Interestingly, no single area of the cortex has been identified as the location for memory storage. In fact, the experimental and pathological evidence suggests that memory storage is dispersed through wide regions of the brain, further supporting the idea that memories are more meaningfully understood as encoded pathways of conduction than as discrete anatomical entities.[2] The temporal lobes of the neocortex, and especially the adjacent hippocampal nuclei, however, have been revealed to be indispensable to memory retrieval.

There is evidence to suggest that specialized types of memory—such as, for example, language memory, motor memory, nonverbal conceptual memory, and experiential memory—are to some degree functionally distinguishable, involving separate encoded systems of centrencephalic integration. Experimental research with individuals suffering from amnesia, for example, has confirmed that procedural memory, involving the learning of motor skills, is physiologically independent of declarative or informational memory. The physiological processes that give rise to conceptualization, however, appear to be fundamentally similar, whether the conceptualization involves procedures, motor skills, abstract ideation, or even emotion. All genres of memory exhibit variable longevity, ranging from momentary to relatively permanent.

Although the particular electrochemical basis for memory is not well understood, the potential scope of memory has proven to be extraordinary. Through the direct electrical stimulation of the exposed brains of conscious patients (under local anesthetic), neurosurgeons have determined that the brain stores deep within the cortex a "stream of consciousness" memory of possibly every experience that comes within the focus of awareness. Experiences that are outside the focus of awareness apparently are not saved in memory. As Penfield states, "One can only conclude that conscious attention adds something to brain action that would otherwise leave no record. It gives to the passage of neuronal potentials an astonishing permanence of facilitation for the later passage of current, as though a trail had been blazed through the seemingly infinite maze of neuronal connections"(Penfield, 1975, p. 75).

According to the model of memory formation hypothesized by Penfield, all types of memory are encoded through a process involving the application of attention. It is, for example, the agency of attention that Penfield suggests must accompany the programming of the automatic sensory-motor mechanism. Once a motor skill has been encoded within the automatic sensory-motor mechanism through the application of attention, however, the automatic mechanism proves more efficient than the conscious attentive mechanism in performance of the skill. And once attention is freed from a specific skill by assumption of that function by the automatic sensory-motor mechanism, attention can be brought to bear on either the further refinement of the skill or the development of supporting or even entirely unrelated skills.

It has been suggested on the basis of the physiological model of brain function that the subjective experience of awareness is caused by the generation of high levels of electrochemical conduction in widespread patterns throughout the cortex. Both volitional motor response and attentive sensory perception—in other words, the volitional and attentive aspects to awareness—evidence substantial generalized and sustained cortical potentials. Awareness will arise, in other words, either as volition prior to motor response or as attention subsequent to sensory stimulation. The specific nature and degree of awareness is presumed to be a function of the spatial configuration and frequency of this centrencephalic neuronal conduction. Mechanisms of memory are triggered by a spatial conformation and frequency of conduction sufficient to be experienced as either attentive or volitional awareness. Memory formation does not appear to be triggered without a contemporaneous experience of awareness.

The physiological model of brain function localizes most aspects of mind within the cerebral cortex, integrated with other bodily processes through a highly complex and pervasive system of centrencephalic integration. Through the propagation of an integrated transcortical pattern of neuronal activity, the brain is able to encode conceptual memory. All forms of memory—for example, motor memory, language memory, experiential memory, and nonverbal conceptual memory—arise in subjective awareness only as conceptualization. All memory is presumed to be a result of subcellular changes caused by the conduction of neuronal potentials. Although other more subtle adaptations potentially occur in each neuronal mechanism of propagation by virtue of every episode of conduction, only patterns of neuronal conduction that induce a subjective sense of awareness, experienced to some degree as either volition or attention, cause the functionally dramatic molecular changes that physiologically encode conceptual memory. Conceptual memory, then, can be understood to involve the structural facilitation of a specific pattern of centrencephalic conduction caused by a prior conduction in that pattern accompanied by a subjective experience of volitional or attentive awareness. The quality or intensity of the experience of awareness is presumed to be a reflection of the scope, duration, and intensity of the cortical activity. The operation of mind, therefore, is understood to be controlled entirely by the physiological processes of the brain.

The Physiology of Emotion

The subjective experience of emotion characteristically is distinguished from the experiences of mind categorized as conceptual awareness. On analysis, however, this dichotomy of mental experience is revealed to be illusory.

The brain centers most directly associated with emotion are components of what is called the limbic system. The pivotal processing center for the limbic system is believed to be the hypothalamus. The hypothalamus, located immediately adjacent to the midline ventricular system, is closely integrated (through reciprocal projections) with the hippocampus, the amygdala, the septal areas, and the anterior thalamus. The hypothalamus appears to be the central processing body for the sympathetic autonomic nervous system, with executive control over the glands and smooth muscles of the internal organs exercised through projection tracts running to the pituitary complex and to the motor neurons of the autonomic system. With a few exceptions, these latter efferent projections are interrupted, frequently on multiple levels and most notably by processing interchanges within the reticular formation.

Afferent projection tracts originating in proprioceptors insinuated in the autonomic nervous system ascend to the hypothalamus from spinothalamic nerve tracts mediated through interruptions within the reticular formation. The hypothalamus, in turn, appears to be integrated intimately with virtually the entire neocortex through parallel projection tracts connecting the cortical areas with the temporal lobes, the hippocampus, and the amygdala. It appears likely that the state sensors presumed responsible for regulating the sympathetic autonomic nervous system, located in the midline ventricular area and mediated predominantly by the hypothalamus, project messages relating the state of autonomic arousal to the cortex. In addition, the reticular formation's modulation of cortical tone may be influenced by its processing of afferent feedback from the sympathetic autonomic system. It is probable, therefore, that sensory feedback from the sympathetic autonomic nervous system reaches various regions of the neocortex, conveying "feelings" of variable states of sympathetic autonomic arousal to cortical areas integral to conceptual awareness. These feelings of arousal are then interpreted by the cortical processes, giving rise to awareness in the conceptual terms of emotion—as, for example, love or hate and joy or despair. Investigations of lateralization of functions between the two cerebral hemispheres suggest that those cortical areas most involved in emotion are centered within the right cerebral hemisphere.

It is not incidental, in other words, that those same mechanisms that appear to govern emotion are also central components of the brain mechanisms controlling the sympathetic autonomic nervous system. In fact, emotional feelings can be understood to be a unique genre of sensory perception, reflecting the state of arousal of the sympathetic autonomic nervous system.

Emotions, therefore, can be understood as feelings, but only in the sense that all modes of sensory reception arise as feelings. The somatic exteroceptor mechanisms do quite literally feel an external universe, and the specific receptor organs that give rise to the sensations of vision, olfaction, hearing, and taste all can be interpreted as "feeling" the impact of external stimuli. Yet the exteroceptor and proprioceptor mechanisms of the various sensoria translate these feelings into neuronal codings of impulse frequency and conduction pathway, such that sensory perception manifests within the brain as an electrochemical code. That electrochemical code can only arise in consciousness, however, as a concept. The idea that emotions arise in consciousness as feelings is, then, unobjectionable, but only insofar as those feelings are cast in terms of conceptualization. The feelings of emotions, therefore—whether characterized as, for

example, love, hate, anger, depression, fear, jealousy, sorrow, or joy—
like the feelings of sensory perception, are electrochemical codings that
arise in awareness as concepts. Feelings, in other words, are translated
into thought within the focus of conceptual awareness.

Psychologist George Mandler has developed a model of emotion that
supports this physiological analysis. Mandler suggests that emotion consists of two distinct components: arousal and evaluation. Any interruption
or discrepancy in an individual's expectations produces arousal of the
sympathetic autonomic nervous system, and "it is autonomic arousal that
produces the hot quality, the intensity aspect of emotion." Mandler distinguishes the generalized arousal states triggered by action of the sympathetic nervous system from more localized systems of arousal such as,
for example, those exciting sexual desire. Generally, however, Mandler
observes that "things like joy and love and fear and anxiety, all seem
to have the same global feeling of arousal to them" (Miller, 1983, p. 140).

The evaluational aspect of emotion necessarily implies the translation
of emotional feelings, especially including those sensations related to
autonomic arousal, into conceptual awareness. Evaluation, therefore, consists of the introduction of emotional feelings into conscious awareness
and involves the interpretation of those feelings in normative conceptual
terms. Mandler illustrates the nature of the evaluative aspect of emotion
through an analysis of the origin of those normative standards in terms
of which emotions arise in awareness:

> There are three sources of evaluation, and as a first approximation
> one can think of these values as arrayed on a continuum of good
> things to bad things. The first are innate, genetically established
> sources of value. These are selected by the evolutionary process, and
> they are good and bad events that have been identified as such in
> the history of the species. Then there are the values that are cultur-
> ally acquired, which we learn about as a result of growing up in our
> culture and society. The third kind of value is derived from the struc-
> tural aspects of events, of the way we perceive and become used
> to their internal structure. (Miller, 1983, pp. 144-145)

It is difficult to imagine how such terms or modalities of evaluation differ
from the evaluative modalities employed in general sensory perception
and cognition. Mandler hypothesizes that the peripheral arousal states
associated with emotion "potentiate" the cerebral evaluations, giving rise
to the "feeling" aspect to emotional evaluation. As evidence of the poten-
tiation of the conceptual, evaluative aspect of emotion by autonomic
arousal, Mandler cites the depreciation of emotional life in individuals
suffering from spinal cord injuries that preclude or diminish sensory experience of autonomic arousal (Miller, 1983, pp. 144-147). Moreover, it
can be hypothesized that the illusory distinction between conceptual

awareness and emotional feeling is encouraged by the apparent concentration of emotional perception within the nonverbal right hemisphere. In other words, emotion arises in awareness principally within the right cerebral hemisphere, in which the terms available for conceptualization are far more abstract than those accessible within the left hemisphere through the faculties of language centered there.

The Incorporeal Universe of Conceptual Awareness

The physiological processes of the brain are determined by two distinguishable paths of evolution: genetic and somatogenic. The process of genetic evolution is conceived as fundamentally determinative of individual anatomy and physiology, and this process includes the brain. The unimaginably sophisticated mechanisms that comprise and sustain the basic systems of life all are coded in detail in patternings of four amino acids on the helical framework of the dioxyribonucleic acid (DNA) molecule. This coding, within the conceptual model of genetic evolution, is understood to have evolved from the finite past in a process of causation grounded in random mutation and natural selection. The human body, through the process of genetic evolution, is equipped at birth with incredibly sophisticated systems that permit extremely complex innate physiological functioning. Not only does the newborn human possess exquisite autonomic systems to sustain life, but each individual also possesses elaborate mechanisms that permit the physiological machinery to be supplemented, adapted, and programmed for further and alternate functions.

The life cycle involves the constant and unavoidable adaptation of the genetically encoded physiological processes in response to somatogenic experience. Indeed, each physiological process within the body is to some degree susceptible to somatogenic adaptation. The most direct connections between the internal physiological processes of an individual and an external physical environment are through the systems of digestion, respiration, and sensory perception. The processes of digestion and respiration are extremely potent mechanisms of somatogenic adaptation. The internal environment is potentially transformed in fundamental ways through the food and breath assimilated by these systems. Yet the most immediate and palpable systemic agency for adaptation of internal physiological processes to an external universe is the nervous system. Not only is the nervous system the agency of all sensory perception, but it also exercises executive control over virtually all bodily processes, including the digestive and the respiratory systems.

The vast preponderance of the functions accomplished by the nervous system proceed autonomically or automatically, and do not entail conscious awareness. Yet automatic functions initially are programmed through physiological processes attended by conscious awareness, and even the autonomic nervous processes display some degree of adaptability, and can be conceived to evolve over the life cycle.

The development of the brain involves extremely complicated growth processes that are only beginning to be understood. It appears, however, that the brain does not generate additional or replacement neurons after birth. To the contrary, there is considerable evidence that neuronal proliferation during embryological development achieves a peak population of neurons that then decreases, in some places dramatically, through a process of selective cell death and elimination. However, recent evidence also suggests that the connections between nerve cells can increase or decrease substantially through post-birth developmental processes. The dendritic and axonal extensions that interconnect neurons are subjected to processes of both selective elimination and proliferation. For example, experimentation on animals—principally rats—subjected to controlled sensory deprivation during rearing, reveals that the cortex actually thickens in long-term developmental response to stimulation. Pribram elaborates:

> *Detailed histological analysis of the thickened cortex showed—as would be expected because neurons do not multiply after birth— that the number of nerve cells per unit volume actually decreased slightly. An increase in the number of branchings of basal dendrites, neurons that extend their fibers horizontally in the cortex, has, however, been reported as has an increase in the number and distention of dendritic spines, small hairlike protrusions on dendrites which are presumed active junctional sites. But a large part of the thickening resulted from an increase in non-neural cells—the glia.* (Pribram, 1981, p. 32; see Figure 14)

Pribram goes on to suggest that similar processes of neural and glial growth continue throughout life and are responsible for the formation of memory. Changeux also suggests a process of dramatic postnatal neuronal development, or "epigenesis," that involves the "selective stabilization of synapses":

> *A remarkable feature of the development of the human brain . . . is that it continues long after birth. . . . As we have seen, brain weight increases by a factor of 4.3 up to adulthood. Most of the synapses of the cerebral cortex are formed after birth. The fact that synapses continue to proliferate postnatally permits a progressive 'impregnation' of the cerebral tissue by the physical and social environment.* (Changeux, 1985, p. 242)

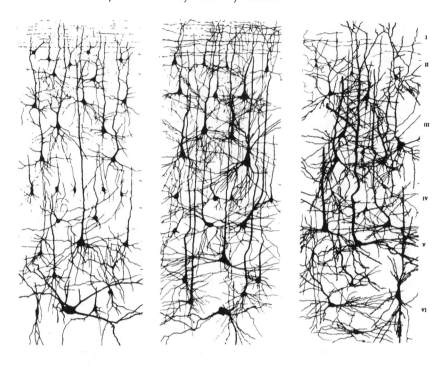

Figure 14. Golgi-stained nerve tissue from the superior temporal cortex in infants aged three months, fifteen months, and twenty-four months, showing the proliferation of dendritic branches in cortical neurons as the infant ages. *Note.* From *Neuronal Man: The Biology of Mind* (p. 199) by J.-P. Changeux, translated by L. Garey, 1985, New York: Pantheon. Adapted by permission.

The most profound somatogenic adaptations involve this lifelong process of encoding conceptual memory within the central nervous system. Conceptual memory is structurally encoded through subcellular molecular adaptations within the pathways of centrencephalic conduction. The necessary precondition for the physiological encoding of conceptual memory is presumed, within the physiological model, to involve organic cerebral processes that are subjectively experienced as awareness in the form of either volition or attention. Conceptual memory, therefore, is encoded through processes that arise in consciousness simultaneously as conceptualization and awareness but that are ultimately presumed to be the consequence of organic brain function. Yet the physiological processes that give rise to conceptualization thereby create an incorporeal universe of abstraction distinguishable from the physical realm of matter and energy. Highly sophisticated conceptual systems of association and differentiation between concepts evolve as language, logic, culture, complex coordination, and the like. This incorporeal universe involves the abstraction and conceptualization of order within the material universe, including the conceptualization of laws of relationship governing the phenomenal universe of matter and energy in space and time. Even models of the physiology of mind exist preeminently as relationships within this intangible realm of abstraction.

The incorporeal universe of conceptualization therefore is presumed to mirror the physical realm of matter and energy in space and time. Because conceptualization arises always in awareness, either as volition or attention, each specific subjective experience of awareness is conceived to correlate precisely with a specific, underlying physiological process of memory encoding. Awareness in either aspect, volition or attention, arises in all shadings of specificity and intensity of focus. In the Physiological Model of Mind, these shadings precisely reflect the specificity and intensity of the cerebral processes that give rise to conceptualization.

Notes

[1]Sensory receptors are classified as either "exteroceptors," which respond to stimuli that originate outside the body, or "proprioceptors," which respond to stimuli arising within the body.

[2]The most famous experimental inquiry into the localization of memory was performed by Karl Lashley, whose search for memory stores, or "engrams," within the brain concluded with his cynical declaration of failure and frustration: "I sometimes feel, in reviewing the evidence on the localization of the memory trace, that the necessary conclusion is that learning just is not possible at all. Nevertheless, in spite of such evidence against it, learning does sometimes occur" (quoted in Pribram, 1981, p. 26).

6

An Empirical Model of the Phenomenal Universe: The Theory

The universe is made of stories, not of atoms.

Muriel Rukeyser

The Physiological Model of Mind developed in chapters 4 and 5 identifies the brain as the substrate of mind. Transcortical arcs of neuronal conduction, termed *hyperneuronal arcs*, have been hypothesized to give rise to the experience of subjective awareness. The physiological microsystems that produce the hyperneuronal arcs of awareness involve complex electrochemical processes that transpire on a molecular and a submolecular level. It is, then, these fundamental electrochemical processes that are posited as the basis for subjective awareness.

The Physiological Model of Mind does not hypothesize a causal role for the mind in the mechanistic electrochemical processes on which it is grounded. Although the mind is understood to arise as an epiphenomenon attendant on the hyperneuronal arc of awareness, the electrochemical processes of the hyperneuronal arc are conceived to transpire without influence or causative effect from the mind. In other words, the model of mind developed in chapters 4 and 5 appears to be incompatible with the concept of practice, which necessarily involves the potent exercise of the willpower of the mind.

In order to reach a definitive determination of whether the mind ultimately has any effect on the brain, the laws governing the electrochemical processes of neuronal conduction must be identified and analyzed on their most fundamental level. The quest for these most basic physical laws leads to the atomic and subatomic realms and into the discipline of physics.

In many respects, physics constitutes the penultimate expression of the Western path to knowledge. Physics attempts to distill fundamental laws of cause and effect through an analysis of patterns manifest in the empirical measurements of objects and processes within the phenomenal universe. Physics, in other words, attempts to fashion an objective Empirical Model of the Phenomenal Universe. This chapter focuses on whether the fundamental laws of cause and effect that underpin the Empirical Model of the Phenomenal Universe leave room for original acts of mind. Put differently, the question is whether the Western path to knowledge is irrevocably committed to a rigorously deterministic and mechanistic conception of reality, thereby foreclosing the existence of the willpower of the mind as an original causal force.[1]

The Quest for an Empirical Model of the Phenomenal Universe

> So that how it can be that a stone, a plant, a star, can take on the burden of being; and how it is that a child can take on the burden of breathing; and how through so long a continuation and cumulation of the burden of each moment one on another, does any creature bear to exist, and not break utterly to fragments of nothing: these are matters too dreadful and fortitudes too gigantic to meditate long and not forever to worship.
>
> James Agee

Traditionally, the discipline of physics has embodied an unwavering commitment to a strictly mechanistic and deterministic conception of the phenomenal universe. The classical physics of Sir Isaac Newton, codified during the 17th and 18th centuries, attempted to explain all of physical reality in terms of a few fundamental laws of interaction between matter in motion. Newtonian physics viewed energy as a property of matter, as reflected in the motion of matter. This bifurcation of the phenomenal universe into matter and motion and the subsequent derivation of fundamental laws of material interaction proved for many years to be an extremely reliable and durable model of physical reality.

As the sophistication of the instruments available for measuring the physical universe evolved, the mechanistic conception of classical physics began to show weaknesses. The principles and mathematics of traditional Newtonian mechanics were stretched to accommodate the new experimental findings, but finally they could be stretched no further. The first real failure of Newtonian physics came in the latter half of the 19th century with the inability of classical principles to explain the newly discerned dynamics of electromagnetic conduction. Newtonian mechanics conceived of energy as a property of matter, but electromagnetic waves could be explained only in terms of electrical and magnetic energy fields. Although these energy fields were considered to be properties of a material plenum, called an ether, the new theoretical model of electromagnetic conduction required no such material carrier field for the energy.

The death knell for classical physics was sounded near the beginning of the 20th century with the identification and measurement of a minimum unit of energy, which was called a "quantum." The quantum was conceived to be a minimum action variable within the phenomenal universe. Accordingly, all physical events were hypothesized to occur in action increments that were multiples of, and no less than, the quantum.

The concept of a minimum action variable had profound implications. For almost a quarter century following the enunciation of the theory of the quantum, physicists groped with these implications. Perhaps the most fundamental question related to the identification of a minimum action variable was whether that quantum variable represented matter or whether it represented energy. This fundamental issue became a focal point for theoretical physics through most of the 20th century.

In 1905, Albert Einstein breathed new life into classical physics with the simultaneous publication of three major papers. First, Einstein's explanation of the photoelectric effect hypothesized the existence of quanta called photons as the fundamental ingredients of electromagnetic radiation. Einstein's theory of the photoelectric effect characterized the photon as a massless particle traveling at the speed of light. Electromagnetic waves, therefore, were conceived to be concentrations of photons in direct proportion to the intensity of the electromagnetic radiation.

Second, Einstein published a paper explaining the apparently random motion of particles in suspension, termed Brownian motion, as a product of the unanalyzable collisions between those particles and the smaller particles comprising the medium of suspension. The importance of Einstein's theory of Brownian motion consisted of its extension of classical mechanics to explain apparently random interactions.

Einstein's third paper was his most famous and consisted of his enunciation of the special theory of relativity, which was a consummate accommodation of the then-apparent inadequacies of empirical measurement and scientific objectivism. Indeed, the special theory of relativity reflects the supreme importance of measurement in empirical investigation. All empirical knowledge concerning an objective phenomenal universe is based on measurement. Measurement is the placement of an object or event in space and time through the application of measuring rods and clocks. A valid and replicable measurement, however, requires that the measurement rod or clock occupy the same frame of reference as the object or event to be measured. The special theory of relativity sets forth mathematical equations that permit the reconciliation of two distinct frames of reference that are moving in uniform translation relative to each other. In other words, the theory provides a mechanism through which the frame of reference of the observer/measurer can be adjusted mathematically to coincide with the frame of reference of the object or event to be measured, thereby standardizing and validating the measurement.

Einstein's special theory of relativity was accompanied by a short paper that enunciated his astounding equivalency theorem: $E = mc^2$ (i.e., energy = mass $\times$ the square of the speed of light). This elegant mathematical formalism embodies perhaps the most profound philosophical revelation within the Western empirical tradition. Quite simply, the equivalency theorem describes the interchangeability (i.e., the "equivalency") of matter and energy.

Approximately 10 years after publication of the special theory of relativity, Einstein published his general theory of relativity, which provides a mathematical framework for reconciling measurement processes involving two frames of reference that are accelerating relative to each other. Among the most profound implications of the general theory of relativity is the proposition that the fundamental parameters of measurement—that is, the three dimensions of space and the dimension of time—have no absolute, definite existence. Instead, space and time exist only as properties of a particular "field" of measurement. Any valid process of measurement, then, requires the congruence of the field of measurement belonging to the observer/measurer and the field of measurement associated with the object or event to be measured. With the enunciation of the general theory of relativity, empirical knowledge was understood to be no more than the coincidence of a subjective field of measurement—that is, the field of measurement of the measurer/observer—and an objective field of measurement—that is, the field of measurement of the object or event measured.

Einstein unsuccessfully attempted to extend field theory to encompass and explain virtually all aspects of the phenomenal universe. No matter how it was construed, however, the concept of a field did not resolve the persistent question of whether elementary quantum processes consist of energy waves or of matter. Quanta such as the photon were perceived to exhibit characteristics of both waves and particles depending on the experimental protocol utilized, and theorists struggled to reconcile this apparently inconsistent data.

In 1925, a new mathematical model of the atomic and subatomic domains was proposed. This mathematical theory has been named quantum mechanics, and it has had resounding repercussions within the disciplines of both physics and philosophy. For some time following the publication of the quantum wave relations that comprise quantum mechanics, physicists grappled with the philosophical implications of the equations. Eventually, the quantum wave relations were understood to represent the probability that a particular quantum particle possesses particular physical measurements in time and space. Quantum mechanics, in other words, was interpreted not as an exact physical description of the quantum universe but rather as a statistical expression of probability distributions concerning the fundamental physical properties of individual quanta. The quantum domain, therefore, no longer was understood to be populated by either particles or waves. It became instead the domain of probability.

The Philosophical Implications of Quantum Theory

No physical theory can do more than this: it can describe a physical system only by describing its propensities, from the point of view of physical theory; and it is only a certain metaphysical view which sees them differently—perhaps as regions of space which are, temporarily, packed 'full' of something, and indivisible.

Karl Popper

The extraordinary significance of the theory of quantum mechanics was only gradually understood. Eventually, however, the profound philosophical implications of the theory were articulated almost simultaneously by Werner Heisenberg and Niels Bohr. Heisenberg's *uncertainty principle* and Bohr's *principle of complementarity* coalesced into the *Copenhagen interpretation* of quantum mechanics, and this interpretation enjoys wide acceptance among theoretical physicists even today.

Heisenberg's uncertainty principle mathematically establishes that the fundamental properties of quanta cannot be measured with present precision. The very process of perceiving and measuring any physical property within the quantum domain will alter that property in unpredictable and unanalyzable ways. The process of measurement therefore changes the object or event measured so that it is no longer as it was when measured. More precisely, the uncertainty principle establishes that the fundamental properties of quanta are measurable only relative to one another and that the precision of measurement of one such fundamental physical property requires a reciprocal impreciseness of measurement with respect to the corresponding physical property in terms of which the first property must be measured. Ultimately, therefore, the physical properties defining quanta cannot be given a sharp, present measurement.

Bohr's principle of complementarity also recognized that the fundamental properties of the quantum domain can be defined only relative to one another. Because each fundamental physical property of the quantum level is paired with a complementary property in terms of which it is defined and measured, the precision of measurement for any single property of the quantum domain requires a reciprocal imprecision with respect to the measurement of the complementary property.

The uncertainty principle and the principle of complementarity identify the ultimate limits to empirical measurement. There are two aspects to the failure of measurement. First, as the uncertainty principle reveals, every act of measurement within the quantum domain involves an interaction between the observer/measurer and the object or event measured that changes both observer and object in unanalyzable and unpredictable ways. The act of measurement itself invalidates the present measurement.

Second, the standards of measurement—that is, the measurement rods and clocks—cannot be calibrated for the quantum domain with any definiteness or precision. Measurement becomes entirely relativistic because the measurement standards can be calibrated only relative to the objects or events to be measured. Put differently, each elementary physical property can be measured only relative to a complementary physical property that, in turn, can be measured only relative to that prior physical property it is used to measure.

The fundamental limitations on classical measurement systems within the quantum domain result from the acceptance of the indivisible quantum as a minimum action variable. All measurement processes are, in essence, experimental systems. More specifically, "the very word 'measure' has come to denote mainly a process of comparison of something with an external standard" (Bohm, 1983, p. 121). On the classical level, measurement processes are conceived to subject the properties of matter and events to "indefinite analyzability" (p. 73). This presumption of precision in measurement is a product of the potential application of external standards or units of measurement that are "vanishingly small" in comparison to the property to be measured. The space-time coordinate systems that constitute the common, essential conceptual framework for physical measurement, therefore, must be conceived to be comprised of adjacent points "which differ by an indefinitely small amount" (Einstein, 1952, p. 90). With the acceptance of the quantum as an indivisible elementary action variable, however, the variables separating adjacent coordinate points—that is, the units of physical measurement—no longer can be treated as indefinitely small. Instead, they are bound by some minimal "size" of physical existence: the quantum. In other words, the points on the space-time coordinate grids necessarily become discontinuous.

Measurements placing an object or event in space and time involve the relationship of the object or event to some external standard. That standard is seen to possess a minimal "size," which is presently understood to be the quantum. The most precise measurements conceivable, therefore, must be made in terms of this minimal standard of measurement. Yet there can be no finer external standard in relation to which this most basic, minimal standard of measurement can itself be measured. It can be measured only in terms of its relationship to measuring rods and clocks that are themselves defined (i.e., measured) in terms of the quantum. Ultimately, then, all measurements are relative and indefinite.

Measurements within the quantum domain, then, are devoid of any objective reality. The quantum can be measured only in terms of its equivalence with another quantum, thereby trivializing the measurement in the same way any concept is trivialized by its definition entirely in terms of itself.

An attempt to escape the inherent limitations of measurement through comparisons that are expressed in terms of fractions rather than multiples of some measurement standard is no more successful. Certainly, the quantum can be described and "measured" as a fraction of some larger standard, yet that larger standard must ultimately owe its measurement to the quantum. The reciprocal complementarity of measurement processes—that is, their ultimate relativity—is inescapable. Just as measurements expressed as multiples of a minimal unit become meaningless when that measurement standard finally reaches zero, so too do measurements expressed as fractions of some maximal unit become meaningless when that measurement standard reaches infinity.

This understanding of the ultimate relativity of measurement is foreshadowed within Einstein's special and general theories of relativity. To be sure, the absolute relativity of the phenomenal universe, implicit in Bohr's principle of complementarity, differed in important respects from the relativity Einstein had formalized in the special and general theories of relativity.[2] Einstein's special theory of relativity was an incorporation and extension of the principles and laws of classical Newtonian physics to all non-accelerated frames of reference expressed through transformational equations. The general theory of relativity, in turn, was an incorporation and extension of special relativity to accelerated frames of reference expressed through a non-Euclidean field geometry. In retrospect, however, Einstein's theories of relativity can be interpreted on a deeper philosophical level to have pierced the veil of a definite, objective, precisely measurable phenomenal universe.

When Newtonian mechanics is extended to its limits through the application of the special and general theories of relativity, the coordinate system employed as the conceptual framework of space and time ceases to have "the least direct physical significance" (Einstein, 1952, p. 94). Instead, a given set of coordinates defining some body of reference in space and time becomes significant only relative to its coincidence with some other set of coordinates defining another body of reference in terms of which that first body might be measured. Measurement processes, in other words, that provide the terms of cognition within the space-time continuum are inescapably relativistic in operation. Einstein's theory of the equivalency of mass and energy—derived from his special theory of relativity and formalized in the elegant equation $E = mc^2$—brings this implicit recognition of the unavoidable relativity of measurement processes to a theoretical climax of staggering implications.

The concept of mass is fundamental in physical theory. Mass is the quantity of matter a body possesses. Subsidiary concepts such as inertia, weight, and density are all expressed in terms of mass. The equivalency of mass and energy amounts, then, to an equivalency of matter and energy. Einstein's equivalency theorem can be interpreted, in other words, to suggest that matter and energy are fundamental complementary concepts. In fact, the different pairs of complementary properties Heisenberg and Bohr identify can be interpreted as subsidiary to the all-encompassing, archetypical complementary concepts of matter and energy.

The concept of energy, lacking any measurable corporeality, traditionally has been defined exclusively in terms of matter. Classical physics is predicated on the notion that properties of matter are directly perceptible and cognizable, whereas energy has been defined entirely in terms of its effect on such directly discernible properties. The concept of energy, in other words, evolved as a fiction contrived to explain the motions of a universe of matter. Eventually, however, the fiction entirely consumed the reality. Energy relations between elementary particles were cast in the form of fields of wave motion until the wave field became indistinguishable from the particle. And finally, with the mathematical formalisms of quantum mechanics, process and object were merged in wave forms of probability. The putative reality of matter that gave rise to the fiction of energy ultimately was recognized as a fiction itself, being contrived entirely in terms of processes and patterns of energy relations. Einstein's formalism describing the interconvertability of matter and energy therefore presaged the contemporary probability formulations that posit both matter and energy in wave form.

In essence, the relativity relationship defines two complementary concepts in terms of their relative displacements from an intermediate state of dynamic equilibrium. That state of dynamic equilibrium, however, is defined reciprocally in terms of the equal and opposing displacements of the two complementary concepts. At its most fundamental level, relativity theory locks perception and cognition into a framework of reciprocity and mutual reification that presumes and guarantees order and internal consistency in conceptualization.

The Copenhagen interpretation of quantum mechanics also suggests that an objective world of definite physical phenomena does not exist except in relation to an observing consciousness. Again, Einstein's theories of relativity anticipated this philosophical interpretation of quantum mechanics. And again, Einstein demurred from such conclusions, insisting that the scientific observer could be conceptually isolated from the event observed.

Both the special and the general theories of relativity are concerned principally with reconciling distinct frames of reference in motion relative to each other. Einstein speaks in terms of bodies of reference, which he describes mathematically within the conceptual framework of Galileian (now commonly referred to as Cartesian) space-time coordinates for special relativity and Gaussian space-time coordinates for general relativity. Any single set of coordinates, however, can be meaningful only relative to some other set that operates as measuring rod or clock. That measurement body of reference therefore must be attuned to the frame of reference of the observer/measurer. For this reason, the measurement process is invested with meaning only by virtue of the observer's participation. In other words, Einstein's relativity theories provide the conceptual framework within which the distinct frames of reference of the observer and the event observed can and must be integrated. Physical concepts, to be meaningful, must involve measurements of time and space that bind the observer and the phenomenon observed within a single physical system.

A closer look at the statistical basis of quantum mechanics is necessary to understand the putative departure from classical notions of a deterministic universe. According to quantum theory, individual phenomena within the atomic domain occur at random. Randomness is, in fact, the exclusive conceptual category within physics that escapes the encompassing reach of determinism. It is critical to note, however, that the concept of randomness has no affirmative, substantive meaning, for to define randomness would be to describe what must remain beyond description (see Pagels, 1982, p. 102). Both mathematicians and physicists, therefore, maintain an operational approach to definitions of randomness and probability. Randomness, consequently, is defined as the independent fluctuation of contingencies outside a given causal context in an unanalyzable way over a wide range of possibilities ''but in a manner that statistical averages have a regular and approximately predictable behavior'' (Bohm, 1984, p. 22). Randomness, therefore, loses all absolute meaning and becomes definitionally dependent on the depth and focus of analysis by a perceiving consciousness. Bohm underscores this point with his observation that ''just as a causal law can arise as a statistical approximation to the average behavior of a large aggregate of elements undergoing random fluctuations, a law of chance can arise as a statistical approximation to the effect of a large number of causal factors undergoing essentially independent motions'' (p. 143). Therefore, Bohm suggests ''that the possibility of treating causal laws as statistical approximations to laws of chance is balanced by a corresponding possibility of treating laws of probability as statistical approximations to the effect of causal laws" (p. 65). In other words, the processes of perception and cognition themselves entirely determine whether a phenomenon will be conceived as the product of causal laws or of laws of chance—that is, as the product of determinism or of randomness.

Consequently, Bohm argues that the forfeiture of causality on the quantum level, although operationally acceptable, need not have absolute significance. "Hidden variables" operating on a subquantum level conceivably could be causally determinative of individual quantum phenomena without disrupting the apparent randomness of such phenomena to our systems of observation. An entirely new system of observation and measurement must be postulated in order to avoid the conclusions of quantum indeterminacy inherent in Heisenberg's uncertainty formulation if the hypothetical subquantum level of hidden variables is to be probed further. Moreover, even the hidden properties to be observed and measured must be fundamentally distinct from the quantum mechanical "observables" understood within quantum theory to fluctuate at random and to be exclusively complementary for purposes of measurement. In essence, Bohm (1984) suggests that the subquantum level may be qualitatively distinct from the quantum level, possessing relatively autonomous properties and relationships (pp. 50-51). He does not propose that all subquantum variables can be determined to unlimited accuracy any more than variables of the quantum level can be so precisely determined. However, Bohm (1983) does suggest that through experimentation one might be able "to show that the sub-quantum level is there, to investigate its laws, and to use these laws to explain and predict the properties of higher-level systems in more detail, and with greater precision, than the current quantum theory does" (p. 121).

It is important to emphasize that the revelation of hidden variables within a subquantum domain would have the effect only of reducing the size of the quantum units of perception and measurement utilized within the conceptual system. It would not abrogate the ultimate necessity for elementary quantum units of cognition. Our capacity for perception and measurement on the microscopic level is limited by the "size" of the quantum unit employed to relate that microscopic level to the macroscopic level of sensory perception. Quantum mechanics operates on the assumption that the minimum action variable for the atomic domain is the quantum. Should, as Bohm suggests, a smaller action variable be operant on a subquantum level, then the possibility arises for utilizing that smaller unit as a standard to perceive and measure the quantum domain with greater precision than Heisenberg's uncertainty formulation would permit. However, uncertainly would not be eliminated but only removed to the next deeper level of analysis.

The Copenhagen interpretation of quantum mechanics is by no means universally accepted. There are a number of theorists who believe, with

Bohm, that the imprecision of measurement on the quantum level is only a reflection of temporary (though formidable) limitations on our instruments and techniques of measurement. Eventually, they hypothesize, the apparent indeterminacy of the quantum domain will be revealed to be determined according to the mechanistic physical laws operating within a subquantum domain. Yet, even if a subquantum domain with a lesser action variable is hypothesized to exist, the end of measurement would be only one step further removed from the classical level. Ultimately, there must always be some "thing"—some minimal standard of measurement that is greater than nothingness—in terms of which measurements may be made. If it is not the quantum, it still must be some lesser "thing."

The result of these ultimate limitations on measurement is that physics becomes on the quantum level—or on whatever subquantum level is determined as minimal—predominantly instrumental rather than conceptual. Bohm (1984) summarizes this fall from grace: "Thus, it is concluded that conceptual thinking will be restricted to the classical domain only, while outside this domain the only thing left to do will be to engage in purely technical manipulations of mathematical symbols according to suitable prescriptions which it is the business of theoretical physicists to discover" (pp. 96-97).

Our knowledge will not, then, be saved from the uncertain realms of probability theory by instruments of greater precision and resolution that assist the senses in probing the frontiers of the large and small. There is, rather, an inherent flaw in the process of perception itself; or, to put it another way, the process of perception, like all conceptualization, is limited. Beyond knowing is not-knowing, a realm that is entirely inaccessible to the processes of human awareness. It is, like the concepts of infinity and nothingness, ultimately beyond naming or describing except in terms of what it is not.

The Limits of Cognition

> For the only way one can speak of nothing is to speak of it as though it were something.
>
> Samuel Beckett

The theory of quantum mechanics, replete with the Copenhagen interpretation, has had a profound philosophical impact. Yet in retrospect it is clear that both the absolute relativity and the nonobjectivity of the phenomenal universe were suggested by Einstein's consummate extensions and accommodations of a classical physics committed to a definite and objective physical reality. A close analysis of the philosophical implications of quantum physics, however, reveals that the qualities of absolute relativity and nonobjectivity need not inhere in the phenomenal universe presumed to exist separate and apart from an observing consciousness. In fact, the claim that quantum mechanics requires a forfeiture of the concept of determinism within the atomic domain is not accurate.

Ultimately, a deterministic conceptual framework is indispensable to Western empiricism at all levels of analysis. What must be abandoned at the quantum level is the possibility of making any deterministic laws accessible to human observation and meaningful measurement. Heisenberg's uncertainty principle requires that, so long as the minimum action variable is the quantum, quantum properties will remain inaccessible to definitive measurement. Bohr's principle of complementarity suggests that quantum properties exist in complementary pairs and that we are prevented from simultaneously measuring both complementary properties. Neither theorist rejects quantum level determinism per se but only determinism relative to an observing consciousness.

Even the very existence of an external physical reality—external, that is, to consciousness—can be established and verified only through and to an observing consciousness. Yet the theory of quantum mechanics implies that the processes of observation and measurement that might verify the existence of a definite, objective reality external to consciousness are fundamentally and irremediably flawed. In other words, a definite, objective, external universe may indeed exist, but an observing consciousness can know it only as an act of faith, and never through acts of measurement or experimental proof.

The Copenhagen interpretation of quantum mechanics suggests that the limitations on the possibilities of verifying the existence of a definite, objective, external quantum world inhere in the processes of observation and measurement. Those processes, however, are nothing more than an extension of the observing consciousness and its conceptual framework for perception and comprehension. The processes of observation and measurement, in other words, are entirely determined by the framework of cognition constituting the observing consciousness: *adaequatio rei et intellectus*. If, as the Physiological Model of Mind suggests, the observer is limited to a binary framework of conceptualization in which concepts arise and decline always in complementary reciprocity, then the complete relativity of the phenomenal universe will be the observer's inescapable perception regardless of whether the phenomenal universe is definite and objective or completely relative and observer created. Or, put more simply, any conceptualization of an absolute, unique, and objective reality will itself be preeminently a mental phenomenon that is both observer created and completely relative. Any deeper analysis of reality must abandon the conceptual process entirely to avoid the cognitive framework of complementary reciprocity. And, or course, analysis is impossible without conceptualization.

The Copenhagen interpretation of quantum mechanics, therefore, suggests that our empirical knowledge of the phenomenal universe must remain, ultimately, absolutely relative and imprecise. It bears reiteration, however, that these fundamental limitations on measurement relate to the human processes of cognition and not necessarily to an objective physical reality. It is a mistake, therefore, to assume that the uncertainty principle and the principle of complementarity require the forfeiture of the mechanistic, or deterministic, conception of the phenomenal universe. The universe may or may not be an entirely deterministic mechanism. The Copenhagen interpretation of quantum mechanics simply establishes that the measurements that would confirm or refute determinism are inaccessible to human cognition. Therefore, although an objective, measurable phenomenal universe may exist external to an observing consciousness, that consciousness can know the objective universe only as an act of faith. Acts of empirical proof must rely on measurement, and measurement ultimately must remain entirely relativistic and imprecise. The recognition that the quantum realm is cognizable only in terms of probability is not necessarily a statement about the quantum realm or about an objective physical reality generally but is rather a profound commentary on the cognitive processes themselves.

There have been, then, two interpretations of the mathematical formalisms of quantum mechanics. The majority of physicists have been persuaded by the principles of uncertainty and complementarity underlying the Copenhagen interpretation of quantum mechanics. Accordingly, most theoretical physicists adhere to the idea that the minimum action variable accessible to cognition is the quantum and that human consciousness is forever precluded from any precise knowledge of individual events or entities within the quantum domain. To human awareness, the quantum realm is one of randomness and probability, and is substantially beyond the reach of cognition. The wave relations of quantum mechanics, therefore, are interpreted to be probability distributions rather than actual physical descriptions of quantum entities in time and space.

A minority of theoretical physicists have rejected the Copenhagen interpretation as too broad and absolute in its postulates. Instead, these theorists have suggested that the wave equations of quantum mechanics can be interpreted as partial physical descriptions of quantum phenomena. Moreover, they have hypothesized the existence of a subquantum realm of physical reality, in which the elementary unit of cognition (i.e., the minimum action variable) is less than the quantum. The concept of a subquantum domain does not violate the principles of uncertainty and complementarity. Rather, it suggests that these principles are limited to the quantum level of the phenomenal universe. Within the subquantum level of reality, qualitatively different laws of interaction are hypothesized to govern the rise and decline of properties not cognizable on the quantum level.

Ultimately, human consciousness cannot pierce through all levels of existence—macroscopic, cellular, molecular, atomic, quantum, subquantum, ad infinitum—to reach an ultimate, absolute empirical understanding of the physical universe. The processes of cognition can be pursued in the direction of the vanishingly small, just as they can reach toward the infinitely large. Yet cognition stops, absolutely and inescapably, with the concepts of nothingness and infinity. However far science is able to thrust the senses into the world of the vanishingly small—whether the limits be found in the quantum, the subquantum, or some further level of minimal existence—still there must always remain some "thingness" to which cognition can be anchored. And at that ultimate level of thingness, which now appears to be the quantum level, cognition will be limited, absolutely and inescapably, by the principles of uncertainty and complementarity or by exact extensions of these principles into subquantum realms.

The realms of abstract mathematical analysis are remote from direct sensory experience and cannot be adequately translated into language. Yet even these lofty realms are limited. The particles of the physical universe become waves in a vibration between matter and energy from one moment of time to the next, and the terms of conceptualization fall from certainty to probability. And in randomness and probability, no less than in nothingness and infinity, the limits of cognition are reached. Beyond is the realm of failure and disorder, beyond limits, empty of conceptualization.

Finally, then, deep within the hidden quantum and subquantum realms, the Western path to knowledge ends. The empirical processes of observation and measurement have proven to be limited. Ultimately, the attempt to fashion an Empirical Model of the Phenomenal Universe also must be limited. The limits are to be found, however, within the cognitive processes themselves and not necessarily within the phenomenal universe.

The fundamental processes of the phenomenal universe have proven to be impenetrable to empirical measurement and cognition. It is therefore impossible to determine with certainty whether the electrochemical processes of neuronal conduction are causally affected by the willpower of the mind. The search for the mind, in short, reaches an impasse at the limits of the Empirical Model of the Phenomenal Universe. This chapter and chapter 7 explain and analyze that impasse. Chapter 8 begins the exploration of the frontier beyond the Western path to knowledge.

Notes

[1]The Empirical Model of the Phenomenal Universe developed in this chapter is derived from a broad sampling of the nonmathematical literature of theoretical physics. Chapter 7 contains a more detailed review of the historical development of contemporary theoretical physics, and the reader is referred to that chapter for clarification and elaboration of the scientific principles and theories that are presented in more summary fashion in chapter 6.

[2]The Copenhagen interpretation of quantum mechanics raised the specter of the complete relativity and nonobjectivity of the phenomenal universe. Not surprisingly, such a profound reordering of fundamental physical and philosophical precepts encountered strong resistance among physicists and philosophers alike. Although Bohr emerged as the principal spokesperson for the Copenhagen interpretation of quantum mechanics, Einstein rose to champion the theoretical opposition to that interpretation. The frequently eloquent and provocative exchanges between Bohr and Einstein never reached a definitive resolution, and the validity of the Copenhagen interpretation remains uncertain. It has, however, won the favor of a majority of theoretical physicists—although some of the discipline's most distinguished practitioners still demur—and its far-reaching philosophical implications have become increasingly palatable over time.

7

An Empirical Model of the Phenomenal Universe: The Evidence

*Now understand me well—It is provided in the essence of things,
that from any fruition of success, no matter what, shall come forth
something to make a greater struggle necessary.*

Walt Whitman

To reach the limits of the Physiological Model of Mind, the level of analysis must descend from the cellular and molecular levels to the atomic and subatomic levels, where matter and energy are conceived in their most elementary forms. Traditionally, this is the realm of physics, in which precise empirical models of the physical universe are articulated as mathematical formalisms. Mathematics constitutes the most powerful Western system of conceptualization available to abstract order from the interplay of matter and energy in space and time that we experience as physical phenomena.

It is, of course, beyond the scope of these writings to provide more than a general and nonmathematical review of classical and contemporary theoretical physics. However, an understanding of modern physics is virtually impossible without some appreciation of its historical development. Consequently, the quest for an Empirical Model of the Phenomenal Universe must begin with an extremely abbreviated chronology highlighting the major themes that have shaped the contemporary discipline of theoretical physics.

Newton: The Entrenchment of Classical Physics

The quest for mathematical order and pattern within the physical universe reached a culmination of sorts in the 17th century with the codification of the mechanistic cosmology in Newtonian physics. All physical phenomena, within Newton's system of conceptualization, were reduced to matter and motion, and specific laws of mechanical interaction were formulated and articulated mathematically to explain the interaction between discrete units of matter. Newtonian mechanics were then successfully extrapolated to explain the behavior of waves, such as sound and light, propagating through some continuous medium of matter.

By the mid-19th century, the application of basic Newtonian mechanics in increasingly sophisticated mathematical formulations seemed adequate to explain all physical phenomena, whether manifest in wave form or particle form. These conceptual models for describing physical phenomena began to fail, however, when confronted with certain fundamental properties exhibited by electricity and magnetism.

Traditional Newtonian mechanics were employed by James Clerk Maxwell in his formulation of a mathematical theory of electromagnetism, but his theory went well beyond the limits of any prior mechanical model. Maxwell's theories rested predominantly on the experimental work of Michael Faraday. Maxwell developed a mathematical model of electromagnetism that accommodated Faraday's burgeoning experimental evidence regarding electrical induction. His mathematical system involved a restatement of the Newtonian concept of force in terms of force fields. Maxwell posited the concept of a field to describe that quality or condition of a region of space that is capable of producing a force. Maxwell, utilizing this mathematical model, then deduced that an electrical field changing in space over time generates a magnetic field and that a magnetic field changing in space over time generates an electrical field. On the basis of this mutually generative relationship between changing electrical and magnetic fields, Maxwell hypothesized that light is an electromagnetic wave propagated through the alternating, serial rise and decline of electrical and magnetic fields. Although even Maxwell realized that his mathematical formulations did not require an ether, or material medium, for propagation of electromagnetic waves, he never expressly abandoned the Newtonian idea that all space is filled with matter in ordered motion. Apparently, Maxwell's theory of electromagnetism was so pragmatically significant that its more abstract theoretical inconsistencies with Newtonian mechanics were virtually ignored, even by Maxwell himself.

The foundation of classical physics, however, began slowly to crumble around the turn of the 20th century. In 1900, Max Planck developed the quantum theory, on the basis of experimental evidence regarding the relationship between heat energy and the frequency of heat radiation. Planck "quantified" a minimum unit of energy released through the process of thermal radiation of atoms. This quantum factor, for which Planck identified a numerical value, became known as "Planck's constant." The quantum theory represented the first real rumblings of a new age in theoretical physics.

Einstein: Revolutionary Retrenchment

In 1905, Einstein revolutionized classical physics with the simultaneous publication of three papers describing his theory of the photoelectric effect, his special theory of relativity, and his kinetic theory of Brownian movement. In his theory of the photoelectric effect, Einstein confronted what has proved to be one of the most persistent problems with which physics has grappled: the simultaneous appearance of light (and other forms of electromagnetic radiation) as both particle and wave. Maxwell's model of electromagnetic radiation as a waveform propagated through alternating electrical and magnetic fields accommodated the experimental evidence confirming the wave characteristics of radiation. This evidence came primarily from the experimental observation that electromagnetic radiation from two point sources will form interference patterns characteristic of wave interaction and superposition. Maxwell's conception of electromagnetic radiation as a waveform, however, could not accommodate the experimental evidence demonstrating the radiation to be corpuscular in nature. This evidence came principally from the photoelectric effect, in which the incidence of electromagnetic radiation on a substance causes the ejection of electrons from that substance. Einstein suggested an ingenious interpretation of this seemingly incompatible experimental evidence.

Einstein's theory of the photoelectric effect demonstrated mathematically that Maxwell's theory of electromagnetism did not demand any material medium for wave propagation. On the basis of Planck's quantum theory of thermal radiation, Einstein suggested that electromagnetic radiation is quantized as photons, or massless particles that travel at the speed of light. In other words, Einstein conceived the wave front of electromagnetic radiation to consist of a concentration of photons directly proportional to the intensity of the radiation. The theory of the photoelectric effect marked a radical extension of the prior conception of light as an electromagnetic wave and was not fully accepted until confirmed experimentally in 1923-1924.

Einstein's special theory of relativity was a brilliant accommodation of the classical laws of physics for nonaccelerated frames of reference moving in "uniform rectilinear and non-rotary motion" relative to each other.

The special theory of relativity was based substantially upon the theoretical analyses of H. A. Lorentz. Not only did Lorentz demonstrate that experimental evidence in electrodynamics and optics necessarily implied the constancy of the velocity of light *in vacuo*, but he also derived a set of "transformation equations," called the "Lorentz transformation," reconciling the laws of electrodynamics, including the constancy of the speed of light, for frames of reference moving in uniform translation relative to each other. In the special theory of relativity, Einstein generalized Lorentz's investigations of electrodynamics, rendering the laws of electromagnetism compatible with Newtonian mechanics.

The conceptual framework utilized to describe the objects and processes of nature within classical physics, called a Galileian (or Cartesian) system of coordinates, consists of the three-dimensional spatial coordinates, arbitrarily labeled x, y, and z, and the single coordinate for time, labeled t. The magnitudes of these four coordinates are determined through processes of measurement by measuring rods and clocks and together define the location of the body of reference in space and time. The special theory of relativity recognizes, however, that the frame of reference from which the measurements defining the Galileian coordinates are taken may be moving in uniform translation relative to the body of reference being measured. In other words, the measuring rod or clock may be in uniform motion relative to the object or event it is meant to measure. The system of equations constituting the Lorentz transformation, however, enables the coordinates defining the measuring rod or clock to be adjusted to coincide with the coordinates of the body of reference being measured. The Lorentz transformation effectively integrates the coordinates of the observer/measurer's frame of reference and the object frame of reference into a single physical system. In the words of Einstein (1952),

> Every general law of nature must be so constituted that it is transformed into a law of exactly the same form when, instead of the space–time variables x, y, z, t of the original coordinate system K, we introduce new space–time variables x', y', z', t' of a coordinate system K'. In this connection the relation between the ordinary and the accented magnitudes is given by the Lorentz transformation. Or in brief: General laws of nature are co-variant with respect to the Lorentz transformations. (pp. 42-43)

The implications of the special theory of relativity are far-reaching and profound. Although the significance of the theory becomes paramount with respect to objects only in extremely rapid motion, it requires that such rapidly moving objects will exhibit a relativistic increase in measurements of mass, a contraction in measurements of length, and an expansion, or dilation, in measurements of time. Perhaps the most profound implication of the special theory of relativity, however, is the principle of the equivalency of mass and energy—$E = mc^2$—which Einstein formulated in a brief paper supplementing the special theory of relativity. The third paper Einstein published in 1905 involved an extension of the statistical mechanics of the kinetic theory of gases to explain the rate of molecular displacement evidenced in Brownian motion. Brownian motion is named for the botanist Robert Brown, who, in 1824, observed that microscopic spore particles suspended in water exhibit incessant and patternless motion without discernible cause. Subsequently, smoke particles suspended in air were determined to exhibit similar constant, irregular, and unexplainable movement. Einstein theorized that such irregular motions are the consequence of collisions between the microscopic spore or smoke particles and the molecules constituting the medium of suspension. Just as the kinetic theory of gases explained gas pressure as the statistical result of the essentially random impact of irregularly moving gas molecules on the walls containing the gas, Einstein explained Brownian motion as the consequence of collisions between the chaotically moving molecules of the medium of suspension and the larger suspended particles exhibiting the Brownian movement. This vindication of an essentially Newtonian analysis of molecular motion presaged a retrenchment of classical physics in the early 20th century. Bohm (1983) describes the significance of Einstein's theory within the classical tradition:

With the discovery of Brownian motion, one obtained phenomena that at first sight seemed to call the whole classical scheme of order and measure into question, for movements were discovered which were what have been called here 'order of unlimited degree,' not determined by a few steps (e.g., initial positions and velocities). However, this was explained by supposing that whenever we have Brownian motion this is due to very complex impacts from smaller particles or from randomly fluctuating fields. It is then further supposed that when these additional particles and fields are taken into account, the total law will be deterministic. In this way, classical notions of order and measure can be adapted, so as to accommodate Brownian motion, which would at least on the face of the matter seem to require description in terms of a very different order and measure. (p. 121)

Einstein's statistical analysis, in other words, was interpreted to be a vindication of the classical deterministic order in the face of the apparent "lawlessness" of Brownian motion. In more general terms, then, Einstein's theory of Brownian motion can be interpreted to demonstrate that "lawlessness of individual behavior in the context of a given statistical law is, in general, consistent with the notion of more detailed individual laws applying in a broader context." (p. 68)

The Particle-Wave Dualism Revisited

The atomist conception of ultimate matter climaxed in 1913 with Bohr's description of atomic structure in terms of a positively charged atomic nucleus with negatively charged electrons orbiting at quantized energy levels. Bohr, working from the atomic model postulated by Ernst Rutherford in 1911, hypothesized that atoms exist in alternate stable energy states that involve specific configurations of negatively charged electrons in orbitals around a positively charged nucleus, and that any variation between two such stable states would involve energy transitions of quantum increments. Bohr utilized calculations from atomic spectroscopy of the energy released through the changes between stable atomic states to develop a model of atomic structure with electron orbitals electromagnetically bound at incremental distances from the nucleus that correlated with the quantity of energy involved in the presumed transition of those electrons from one orbital level to another.

In 1923, Louis de Broglie suggested that Maxwell's wave equations might apply to the behavior of electrons and hypothesized that the wavelength of an electron is equal to Planck's constant divided by its momentum. Experimental verification of this relationship came through the wave patterns generated by the crystalline diffraction of electrons. Moreover, de Broglie's electron wave relation provided an abstract mathematical basis from which standing electromagnetic waveforms could be hypothesized to exist at the same distances from the nucleus as did the quantized electron orbitals Bohr had derived from experimental evidence.

De Broglie's formulations suggested a possible reconciliation between the apparently incompatible interpretations of light as an electromagnetic wave field in the theories of Maxwell and as a particle in Einstein's theory of the photon. The electron, according to de Broglie, was conceived as a definite and measurable particle that exists only in association with a wave field.

The concept of a field arose as a procrustean attempt to stretch the concepts of both wave and particle toward some hybridized synthetic notion that would accommodate each without being limited to either. Initially, the concept of field was premised on the existence of a pervasive material carrier medium (ether) for wave propagation. Although the concept of a material, mechanical ether of contiguous matter was unnecessary to Maxwell's mathematical description of electromagnetic wave propagation, the electromagnetic field Maxwell postulated still was understood to be, in some abstruse way, a state of the ether.

Maxwell's electromagnetic theory, however, conceived in relation to a luminiferous ether at rest, proved ultimately to be incompatible with Einstein's special theory of relativity. The crux of the inconsistency lay in the relativistic requirement of the equivalency of all inertial systems, a condition violated by the absolute and preferred inertial system postulated in the form of an ether at rest. In other words, the *rest state* postulated by Lorentz and others to explain the absence of experimentally measurable characteristics for the ether, became entirely untenable within a conceptual model in which all inertial systems could be measured and described meaningfully only relative to other inertial systems. There is, in short, no meaning to the concept of *at rest* within relativity theory. Given the superiority of the field concept to Newtonian particle mechanics in explaining electromagnetic interactions, the notion that fields are a state of a material carrier medium was supplanted by an understanding of the field as, in the words of Einstein (1952), "an irreducible element of physical description, irreducible in the same sense as the concept of matter in the theory of Newton" (p. 150).

In 1915, Einstein published his general theory of relativity. This theory, which Einstein considered his paramount intellectual achievement, extended the special theory of relativity to accelerated frames of reference by postulating the equivalency of gravitational and inertial forces. In the process, the concept of field underwent yet another radical transformation.

The general theory of relativity posited a system of arbitrary curvilinear coordinates, or Gaussian coordinates, in place of the rectilinear Galileian, or Cartesian, coordinate system employed in special relativity.[1] Einstein demonstrates in the general theory of relativity that the gravitational field potentially invalidates the field coordinates that define position and time directly for purposes of special relativity (see Einstein, 1952, pp. 93-94). The Galileian coordinate system employed in special relativity presupposes the validity of Euclidean geometry in giving definiteness to statements regarding an object's location within a space-time continuum. The Lorentz transformations simply permit the reconciliation of such definite statements of position and time as between frames of reference moving in uniform translation relative to each other.

The Euclidean space-time continuum that was presumed valid for designating Galileian coordinates, however, is premised on the hypothetical existence of rigid and definite measuring rods and clocks "arranged rigidly with respect to one another" (Einstein, 1952, p. 94). Within a gravitational field, however, there can be no rigid reference bodies (p. 59). Consequently, "according to the general principle of relativity, the space-time continuum cannot be regarded as a Euclidean one" (p. 93). Einstein found the non-Euclidean alternative to the Galileian system of coordinates in the mathematical analyses of Gauss and Riemann. On the basis of Gauss and Riemann's investigations, Einstein demonstrated that the Galileian system of coordinates can be generalized to an arbitrary continuum of contiguous points oriented in the four dimensions of time and space in which the magnitude of each point differs from its adjacent points "by an indefinitely small amount" (p. 90). The specification of a single set of Gaussian coordinates, therefore—arbitrarily designated X_1, X_2, X_3, and X_4—has "not the least direct physical significance" (p. 94). Instead, the designation of any set of Gaussian coordinates is meaningful only relative to its intersection with another designated set.

Within the special theory of relativity, the Galileian coordinates were assumed to possess direct physical significance because, through application of the Lorentz transformations, the coordinate system became a standard reference framework relative to which a point could be defined and measured. The Gaussian system of coordinates, however, cannot itself be conceived as a reference body but only as a definite but arbitrary four-dimensional continuum within which a point can be defined exclusively in relation to its intersection with another point. One such point symbolizes the event to be observed and measured, whereas the coincident point represents the measurement rod or clock. In the words of Einstein (1952), "The following statements hold generally: Every physical description resolves itself into a number of statements, each of which refers to the space-time coincidence of two events A and B. In terms of Gaussian coordinates, every such statement is expressed by the agreement of their four coordinates, X_1, X_2, X_3, X_4" (p. 95).

The critical theoretical consequence of the general theory of relativity is the realization that the four dimensions of space and time have no absolute, definite existence but exist "only as a structural quality of the field" (Einstein, 1952, p. 155). According to this conception, the gravitational force determines the time and space configuration that constitutes the structural quality of the gravitational field. Consequently, an object that exhibits deflection or acceleration in its motion is not conceived as attracted by a gravitational force. Instead, the gravitational force manifests as a transformation of space and time relative to which the object's motion can be conceived as uniform and rectilinear.

Einstein's grand vision, never realized, was of a "theory which describes exhaustively physical reality, including four-dimensional space, by a field" (Einstein, 1952, p. 157). During the last 25 years of his life, Einstein unsuccessfully pursued this dream of unification by attempting to reconcile the theories of electromagnetism and gravitation within a single conceptual system based on the interaction of fields.

Because of the extreme level of abstraction and complexity involved in the special and general theories of relativity, the full philosophical ramifications of these theories were not immediately recognized, even by Einstein. In retrospect, the theories of relativity can be interpreted to provide a philosophical foundation for even the Copenhagen interpretation of quantum mechanics. Einstein, however, remained one of the most vigilant critics of this interpretation of quantum mechanics until his death in 1955.

The Birth of Quantum Mechanics

Classical physics, which Einstein had resurrected by the force of his theoretical analyses, had reached a crossroads by 1925. Despite the best efforts by physicists to reconcile wave fields with particles, these two interpretations of elementary processes remained conceptually distinct and even antithetical. In classical terms, particles were understood to be the material corpuscles constituting a physically discernible and measurable universe, whereas fields were conceived as the immaterial energies or forces that determine the incessant motion of such corpuscles. Conceptually, particles could not simultaneously be fields. The photon, however, appeared through experimentation to violate this requirement of exclusivity. It appeared to be at once both particle and wave field. An experimental apparatus designed to determine whether photons are particles invariably would confirm that photons are particles. However, an experimental apparatus designed to determine if photons are waves invariably would confirm that photons are waves. Moreover, even the fundamental distinction of classical physics between matter and energy—to which the particle-wave distinction seemed intimately related—was undermined by Einstein's equivalency formulation for mass and energy.

It had become clear that the wave-particle dualism of elementary physical existence could not be accommodated within traditional Newtonian physics and that some new mathematical model of the atomic and subatomic universe was necessary. Erwin Schrödinger,[2] extrapolating from Maxwell's wave equations describing the electromagnetic characteristics of light and from Planck's quantum theory, formulated a mathematical model for the de Broglie wave properties associated with electrons. This theory, called quantum mechanics, suggested that atomic structure exhibits properties of both wave and particle. The essence of Schrödinger's equations, and of modern quantum theory generally, is now understood to involve the utilization of mathematical wave relations to predict the probability that an elementary particle (in this case an electron) will be found at a particular place at a particular time.

Quantum mechanics did not at first appear to require the abandonment of the classical model of the physical universe. Although elementary particles were described through Schrödinger's equations in the mathematics of waveforms, the Newtonian supposition that all creation is matter in motion remained relatively intact. Schrödinger, for example, suggested as an initial interpretation of his equations that the electron (and all quantum phenomena) are quantum *matter-waves*, representing that illusive hybrid of particle and wave for which physicists long had quested. Such an interpretation, however, could not accommodate the inescapable corpuscular properties of the electron. There was too much wave and too little matter in the quantum equations.

In 1926, Max Born offered a bold new interpretation of Schrödinger's equations. According to Born, the waveforms described mathematically in Schrödinger's quantum mechanics were not conceived as a description or model of physical reality. Rather, the wave relation de Broglie and Schrödinger described for elementary particles was interpreted by Born as a probability formulation governing the likelihood that the individual quantum particle would possess particular physical properties. Specifically, Born hypothesized that the square of the amplitude of the Schrödinger wave equals the probability that the electron exists at that point in space. In other words, Born interpreted Schrödinger's wave equations to be a statistical rendering of probability distributions relating to the fundamental properties of elementary particles. Accordingly, the properties and behavior of individual quantum particles could be predicted only in terms of probability and not with definiteness or certainty. Elementary matter no longer was understood to be either particle or wave; instead, it became an abstract probability.

The full implications of Born's interpretation are best demonstrated by reference to general macroscopic applications of probability theory. Although the outcome of any single roll of a die is patently unpredictable and essentially random, the outcome of a large sampling of rolls can be predicted with an accuracy that increases in proportion to the number of samples. So, for example, the likelihood that any single roll will result in a 5 is one in six (i.e., random) whereas the likelihood that one sixth of all rolls will be 5s approaches certainty as the number of samples approaches infinity. Similarly, an individual electron cannot be described as existing in a single, definite space-time configuration but only in terms of probability distributions derived from the space-time configurations of a large sampling of like particles. On the quantum level, the properties of an individual particle cannot be conceived otherwise than as random. So, for example, the half-life of a radioactive element can be determined with a precision approaching certainty, whereas there is no possible way to predict with any precision greater than randomness when a single atomic nucleus will decay and radiate.

The Copenhagen Interpretation of Quantum Mechanics

Born's interpretation of the Schrödinger equation erupted in controversy within the international physics community. Heisenberg and other prominent theoretical physicists had joined Bohr at the Niels Bohr Institute in Copenhagen, Denmark; and in 1927, almost simultaneously, Heisenberg derived the uncertainty principle, and Bohr enunciated the principle of complementarity. The philosophy underlying these two principles became known as the Copenhagen interpretation of quantum mechanics.

Heisenberg's uncertainty principle was derived directly from the Schrödinger wave equations and therefore has a precise mathematical form. Put simply, the uncertainty relation establishes mathematically that both the position and the momentum (momentum = mass × velocity) of an electron cannot be measured with unlimited accuracy. The greater the precision of measurement with respect to one property, the less precision in measurement there will be with respect to the other property. The same uncertainty relation governs measurements with respect to the energy and time of an atomic event. Essentially, Heisenberg's formulation expresses mathematically the critical integration of the observer and the event observed within the process of observation. The uncertainty formulation recognizes, in other words, that every act of measurement embodied within a process of perception inextricably insinuates the observer into the object to be measured. There is an inescapable and unpredictable exchange of quanta between the observer and the event or object observed.

The process of perception of any physical property, therefore, unavoidably will alter the property perceived in unpredictable ways. The greater the precision of measurement and the smaller the property measured, the greater will be the potential unpredictable alteration of the object or event measured by the act of measurement. When the observer assumes a degree of precision of measurement of a particular physical property, the distinct but relative property in terms of which the measured property is defined simultaneously must be presumed to possess a reciprocal imprecision of measurement. The observer, the process of observation, and the object observed are merged and synthesized within the moment of observation. None can exist in separate and inviolate form outside of that synthesis.

Bohr's principle of complementarity lacked the precise mathematical formalism of Heisenberg's uncertainty principle but was no less profound a conceptual device. Simply stated, this principle required that each object of perception possess complementary properties that can be defined exclusively in terms of each other. Consequently, the perception and cognition of one such property will preclude the simultaneous perception and cognition of the complementary property.

Bohr therefore approached the new quantum reality in terms of "complementary pairs of imprecisely defined concepts" (Bohm, 1984, p. 93). In place of the classical notion that physical properties could be observed and measured with definiteness and unlimited precision, Bohr suggested that pairs of fundamental physical properties at the quantum level—such as particle and wave, position and momentum, and time and energy—could be observed and measured exclusively in terms of each other. Such paired properties consequently exist only in a reciprocal relationship with each other in which the degree of precision in the measurement of one property demands a correlative imprecision in the simultaneous measurement of the complementary property. Bohr's principle of complementarity, moreover, hypothesized that such inherent limitations on the precision and definiteness of fundamental physical concepts are absolutely unavoidable at the deeper levels of analysis such as those involving the quantum or any potential subquantum domain.

On the scale of everyday affairs, the uncertainty principle and the principle of complementarity have little relevance. Yet for scientific or philosophical models that aspire to a fundamental, ultimate understanding of the nature of the phenomenal universe, the significance of the principles of uncertainty and complementarity is profound. These principles do not suggest that eventually humans may possess the power to perceive the external universe with exactitude. To the contrary, they suggest that because our perceptions are based on an interaction—that is, an unavoidable and unpredictable exchange of quanta—between the perceiver and the perceived object, that process of perception is doomed to uncertainty.

Uncertainty and Complementarity Revisited

Conceptually, there are two distinct interpretations of the uncertainty principle and the principle of complementarity. The first interpretation is that neither of the fundamental properties defining the electron in time and space—neither position nor momentum—can be given a mathematical description of sharp, present measurement. One of the two properties can be measured with precision, but the act of measurement changes that property such that the present measurement must differ in some unanalyzable (i.e., random) way from the now-past precise measurement. In other words, the past state of a property is accessible to precise measurement but never the present state of that same property. Heisenberg, for example, recognized that "the uncertainty relation does not refer to the past." Yet this precise knowledge of the past comes at the expense of any precise knowledge of the present. The present becomes a domain of statistical patterns rather than precise measurements. And in relation to the mathematical operations within the quantum domain, "this knowledge of the past is of a purely speculative character, since it can never . . . be used as an initial condition in any calculation of the future" (Popper, 1982, p. 62).

There is a critical distinction, in other words, between the use of the standard method of past, or *retrodictive*, measurement within the macroworld and its use within the quantum domain. On the classical level of the macroworld, the property measured is affected *negligibly* by the measurement operation, whereas on the quantum level each act of measurement significantly and randomly alters the property measured. Consequently, retrodictive measurements have present validity and applicability within the macroworld but are inescapably inexact and statistical in nature within the quantum domain.

The second interpretation of the uncertainty principle is, in a sense, an extension of the first. In order to describe the electron within a space-time coordinate system, both position and momentum must be measured with precision. The first interpretation of the uncertainty principle recognizes that neither property can be given a precise, present measurement. The second interpretation recognizes that because position and momentum must be measured sequentially and not simultaneously using different experimental apparatuses, the two measurements will be out of synch; that is, the first property measured will no longer be as measured at the point at which the second property is measured. Consequently, both position and momentum cannot be determined to unlimited precision even with respect to a single point within the past (i.e., retrodictively). And with respect to the present, the second interpretation of the uncertainty principle simply compounds the first; that is, both position and momentum come to the present only as statistical representations.

Philosopher Karl Popper is one of a number of theorists who reject these two interpretations of the uncertainty principle and the principle of complementarity. Popper emphasizes that retrodictive measurements are no less valid on the quantum level than on the classical level; indeed, Popper points out that such measurements are "standard" and "indispensable, especially for quantum physics" (Popper, 1982, p. 63). Popper is even more vehement in his rejection of the second interpretation of the uncertainty relation. In direct opposition to the prevailing Copenhagen interpretation of quantum mechanics, Popper contends that on the quantum level, as on the classical level, both the position and the momentum of a particle can be measured simultaneously in a single operation. He states that "all measurements of velocities or momenta consist essentially in interpreting measurements of position." That is, two successive measurements of position yield a measurement of momentum, and therefore both position and momentum are precisely and simultaneously measurable at the moment of the second measurement of position. In the words of Popper,

It is misleading to suggest that experiments designed to measure position are exclusive of (or 'complementary' to) experiments designed to measure momentum, while two experiments designed to measure position are not exclusive of each other and always produce the same result. The truth is that two experiments to measure position can also not be combined without producing a third experiment—an experiment in which position is measured twice in succession. And what the theory tells us is that (since the particle 'has' a position) these two experiments, if carried out correctly, will yield compatible results. Similarly, the view that measurements of position and momentum cannot be combined in the same experiment is also mistaken: for as we have seen, all so-called measurements of momentum are in fact high-level theoretical interpretations of what is, upon a somewhat lower level of interpretation, a measurement of position. (Bartley, 1982, p. 155)

The crux of the controversy surrounding the Copenhagen interpretation of quantum mechanics involves the question of whether the electron being measured is treated as a particle or as a *wave packet*. If it is measured as a particle, then both position and momentum can be determined simultaneously and precisely, although only retrodictively. But if the electron is analyzed as a waveform—as it must be within the contemplation of the quantum wave relations—then the measurements of position and momentum become exclusive and complementary. This is because position is a function of the wave amplitude, whereas momentum is a function of the wavelength. The more localized or confined is the amplitudinal representation within the applicable coordinate system, the more precisely determined the electron's position is interpreted to be. However, the more localized is the amplitude, the less precise is the wavelength representation within its applicable coordinate system. According to the mathematical wave relations of quantum mechanics, then, the nature of measurement differs between the quantum and the classical levels. And most physicists seem to agree that simultaneous, precise measurement of both the position and the momentum of an electron is not experimentally possible.

Within the quantum wave relations, position and momentum, time and energy, and other sets of complementary properties, are referred to as *non-commuting observables*. Bohm (1983) explains:

As a simple analysis shows, the impossibility of theoretically defining two non-commuting observables by a single wave function is matched exactly, and in full detail, by the impossibility of the operation together of two overall set-ups that would permit the simultaneous experimental determination of these two variables. This suggests that the non-commutativity of two operators is to be interpreted as a mathematical representation of the incompatibility of the arrangements of apparatus needed to define the corresponding quantities experimentally.

In the classical domain it is of course essential that pairs of canonically conjugate variables of the kind described above shall be defined together. Each one of such a pair describes a necessary aspect of the whole system, an aspect which must be combined with the other if the physical state of the system is to be defined uniquely and un-

ambiguously. Nevertheless, in the quantum domain each one of such a pair, as we have seen, can be defined more precisely only in an experimental situation in which the other must become correspondingly less precisely defined. In a certain sense, each of the variables then opposes the other. Nevertheless, they remain 'complementary' because each describes an essential aspect of the system that the other misses. Both variables must therefore still be used together but now they can be defined only within the limits set by Heisenberg's principle. As a result, such variables can no longer provide us with a definite, unique, and unambiguous concept of matter in the quantum domain. Only in the classical domain is such a concept an adequate approximation. (p. 74)

Quantum theory comes, therefore, to a denial that even retrodictive measurements of position and momentum can be both simultaneous and precise. To admit such a possibility would be to deny the wave properties of the electron in favor of its particle properties, a denial that, among other consequences, would violate the mathematical wave relations describing the quantum domain. As Bohm (1983) explains, "It is evident that according to Bohr's interpretation nothing is measured in the quantum domain. Indeed, in his point of view, there can be nothing to measure there, because all 'unambiguous' concepts that could be used to describe, define, and think about the meaning of the results of such a measurement belong to the classical domain only" (p. 75).

Wave Mechanics

In the wake of quantum theory, wave mechanics has emerged as the favored mathematical model for describing elementary matter. Although it does not necessarily follow that all matter exists in wave form—and, in fact, the Copenhagen interpretation implicitly denies that possibility—such a conclusion is compatible with the conceptual framework of quantum mechanics. Indeed, this interpretation of quantum mechanics has been suggested by various theorists, including Schrödinger and de Broglie, since the original publication of the quantum wave relation. Within these interpretations, Schrödinger's wave equation is characterized as a description of a new type of field. It is hypothesized "that the field acts as a wave, and yet (because of non-linear terms in the equations) shows a tendency to produce discrete and particle-like concentrations of energy, charge, momentum, mass, etc. . . . [and] that the particle-like concentrations are always forming and dissolving" (Bohm, 1984, pp. 120-121). Bohm and others have developed a sophisticated yet admittedly incomplete interpretation of the quantum wave relation as "an objectively real field." Although the complexities of this interpretation are beyond the scope of this inquiry, Bohm explains that "it would lead to a concept of the electron as an entity that was continually fluctuating from wave-like to particle-like character, and thus capable of demonstrating both modes of behavior, each of which would, however, be emphasized differently in different kinds of environment supplied, for example, by different arrangements of laboratory apparatus" (p. 109; see also pp. 111-121). Bohm's interpretation, however, remains a minority view and runs contrary to the majority interpretation of the quantum wave relation as a statistical rendering of probability distributions.

Yet within all interpretations of quantum mechanics, the wave is the fundamental and indispensable model of physical reality. Because of this preeminence of wave mechanics as a descriptive model of the phenomenal universe, it is important to understand certain wave properties.

Not surprisingly, in light of the relativity and complementarity of matter and energy, the properties of wave motion are themselves described in terms of matter in motion. Wave motion involves a patterned displacement of an object from a state of equilibrium. The *amplitude* of a wave is a function of the maximum displacement of the object from the equilibrium state. The *period* of a wave is a measure of the time taken for one full vibration involving an object's pattern of equal opposing displacements from and returns to equilibrium. The *frequency* of a wave is a function of the number of such periodic vibrations per second (i.e., over time). The *wavelength* of a wave is the distance between two points of corresponding phase on consecutive wave cycles. The *speed* of a wave is a product of its frequency and wavelength. There are, therefore, three primary parameters that define a periodic waveform: amplitude, frequency, and wavelength. Frequency and wavelength, however, vary in inverse proportion to one another for a wave traveling at a constant speed and are therefore reciprocally related.

Wave patterns relate to one another in terms of a summation of displacements from equilibrium at any point in space and time. This process of summation is called *superposition*. In its extreme manifestations, two wave crests that intersect in time and space form at their intersection a single wave crest with an amplitude equal to the sum of the two individual wave crests, whereas the intersection of a wave crest and a wave trough of equal and opposing amplitudes will cause the complete cancelation of the waveform at the point of intersection. The principle of superposition is clearly reflected in the phenomenon known as *standing waves*.

Standing waves are patterns of periodic displacement that repeat indefinitely through the reflection of waves within a bounded medium. To sustain a frequency and wavelength over time within a bounded waveform, the reflected waveform must be essentially congruent with the impacting waveform. Were it not, the principle of superposition would cause an alteration in the waveform over time. There is, therefore, a strict correspondence between the length of the bounded medium and the wavelength or frequency of the standing waveform. To form a standing wavelength within established boundaries, one half of the wavelength, or some whole number multiple of this half wavelength, must precisely fit the bounded medium. Because frequency varies in indirect proportion to wavelength for a wave traveling at a constant speed, only certain frequencies of wave motion can sustain a standing wave within a particular set of boundaries. The lowest, or fundamental, frequency capable of sustaining a standing wave within given boundaries is the equivalent of the longest wavelength capable of sustaining a standing wave for those same boundaries. Other specific frequencies of standing waves are possible within the same boundaries, but only as whole-number multiples of the fundamental frequency. For musical waveforms in which frequency corresponds to pitch, such higher-frequency standing waves are called *overtones* of the fundamental tonal frequency. This same basic conception of wave overtones, which vibrate in whole-number multiples of a fundamental wavelength, underpins the concept of quantum resonance that is so integral to modern physics.

The de Broglie application of wave mechanics to the description of electron orbitals was an elegant example of the extension of this concept of standing waves. De Broglie hypothesized that the electron orbital formed a bounded medium the length of which equaled the orbital's circumference. Consequently, for electrons moving at a constant velocity, only certain wavelengths and frequencies of vibration would sustain standing waveforms within a given orbital. Some whole number of wavelengths, in other words, must precisely fit the orbital's circumference. Changes of energy states by electrons, necessarily involving changes in wavelength and frequency, were perceived to require correlative changes in the circumference of the electron orbital. Electrons, therefore, were defined as standing waveforms of specific orbital circumference and corresponding frequency and wavelength. And eventually, all that remained of the electron particle, notwithstanding its measurable mass, was a probability formulation expressed in a quantum wave relation. De Broglie's wave relation provided a mathematical reconciliation of the quantum properties of electrons and formed the theoretical basis for the periodic table of the elements.

Contemporary Quantum Theory

Without question, quantum mechanics has proven to be an invaluable conceptual model for analyzing and manipulating the atomic domain. Technological achievements directly grounded on the mathematics of quantum mechanics have changed the face of the Earth and have opened the heavens to human ambition.

Since its inchoate formulation in 1925, quantum mechanics has evolved substantially. With the assimilation of Einstein's special and general theories of relativity, quantum mechanics became known as relativistic quantum field theory, most elegantly represented by the mathematical formalisms of quantum electrodynamics. Quantum electrodynamics, which applied quantum mechanics to the domain of electromagnetic interactions, emerged in the late 1940s as the first comprehensive relativistic quantum field theory.

The electromagnetic interactions, however, are but one of four distinct genres of fundamental interaction within the phenomenal universe. In addition to the electromagnetic interactions, physicists have identified three additional classes of energy relations: gravitational interactions, strong interactions, and weak interactions. The primary thrust of contemporary theoretical physics is to synthesize these four empirically distinct types of interaction within the single conceptual framework of a *grand unified relativistic quantum field theory*. Substantial progress has been made toward this elusive goal, yet both gravitation and the strong interactions have proven extremely resistant to such unification.

Although the genuine breakthroughs of theoretical physics always have pushed the limits of prediction beyond the existing capacity for experimental verification, such breakthroughs are themselves invariably based on empirical information developed through prior observation and experimentation. Current theoretical efforts at grand unification have evolved directly from the extraordinary empirical investigations of the quantum domain. Indeed, it has been through the efforts of experimental physicists that the weak and strong interactions have been distinguished as unique and independent forces within the physical universe.

With the discovery of the enormous energy of the forces binding the positively charged protons to the neutral neutrons within the nuclei of atoms came the recognition that extremely strong interactions exist between nuclear constituents without implicating the electrodynamic forces that hold the electrons in their orbitals around the nucleus. The nuclear force, in fact, is clearly distinguishable from the force of electromagnetism. It is vastly more powerful—on the order of hundreds of times more powerful—and operates only within an extremely limited range.

In the pursuit of an understanding of the atomic nuclear force, an array of high-energy scattering and detection techniques have been developed. Through the acceleration of charged elemental particles to extreme velocities and the bombardment of atomic nuclei and various other subatomic particles with these highly energized subatomic missiles, researchers have been able to fragment target particles, including atomic nuclei. These fragments then are detected and identified through the particular trail they leave within a bubble chamber or other detection device oriented within an electromagnetic field. Researchers within high energy physics have identified, through these methods, over 200 subatomic particles, most of which exist for only extremely limited time periods before transmuting into other more stable particles, such as electrons, protons, photons, and neutrinos.

The multitude of elementary particles identified through high-energy scattering has been divided into two general classifications: leptons and hadrons. All particles, whether classified as leptons or hadrons, are presumed to be affected by the force of gravity, although the gravitational force acting on atomic particles is weak beyond measurement or detection. In addition, all particles that possess an electrical charge are affected by the force of electromagnetism. The leptons and hadrons, however, are distinguished through their participation in weak and strong interactions, respectively.

The great predominance of elementary particles are hadrons, which display the strong interactional characteristics exemplified in the forces binding the constituents of atomic nuclei. Leptons, on the other hand, interact so weakly that they do not manifest in any bound form but only in subtle influences such as those governing the rate of radioactive decay.

The first major step by theoretical physicists toward a grand unified relativistic quantum field theory was achieved by Stephen Weinberg and Abdus Salam in 1967. Weinberg and Salam reconciled the weak interactions with the electromagnetic interactions, already described comprehensively in quantum electrodynamics, within a single theory called the *electroweak theory*. The conceptual device underpinning this unification of electromagnetic and weak interactions is the concept of *gauge symmetry*, leading to the development of *gauge field theory*. The mathematics of gauge symmetry theory is based on the algebras of Lie group theory and was first applied to theoretical physics by Chen Ning Yang and Robert Mills in 1954.

Gauge symmetry is not an easy concept to grasp. Even on the quantum level, gauge symmetries are not directly perceptible or measurable. Intact symmetries are "hidden," or "confined," within quanta and become observable only when the symmetries are "broken." Any stable physical system possesses some degree of symmetry. In a sense, the system's stability is the symmetry. The process of perceiving and measuring a stable physical system, however, necessarily involves the disruption of that system at each point in space through "local measurement operations." The preservation of the system's symmetry in resistance to the disruptive interaction of the local measurement operations implies interactive forces that give to the physical system its stability (see Pagels, 1982, p. 299). The fundamental quantum conceived to mediate such interactions within the contemplation of gauge field theories is termed a *gluon*.

Theorists have postulated the existence of *weak gluons* as the mediating quanta in weak interactions on the basis of a large body of experimental evidence concerning the weak interactions (e.g., the radioactive decay of atomic nuclei and the disintegration of hadrons into stable particles such as electrons, protons, photons, and neutrinos). These weak gluons, termed *intermediate bosons* W^+, W^-, and Z^x, were detected directly only in 1983 through highly sophisticated proton-antiproton collision experiments.

The unification of the electromagnetic and weak interactions is conceived to manifest only at extremely short distances and, consequently, at extremely high energies. These two genres of interaction, in other words, are unified in a single gauge symmetry at high energies only. At lower energies, that symmetry is broken, or concealed. A fourth boson, called the *Higgs particle*, is hypothesized to mediate the breaking of that high-energy symmetry, but current accelerators cannot generate experimental energies high enough to permit its detection.

Recently, much of the attention of both experimental and theoretical physicists has focused on the attempt to reconcile the strong interactions with the Weinberg-Salam electroweak theory. High-energy collision experimentation has probed the depths of elementary particles and forces in an effort to determine the properties and nature of those particles, termed hadrons, that exhibit the strong interaction. Exhaustive attempts to break hadrons into constituent subhadron particles have failed. Hadrons can be shattered by high-energy collision processes, but all the particles that are formed are still hadrons. The energy of the scattering process is transmuted into mass in the form of new and reborn hadron entities. The collision point in time and space, therefore, can be conceived as a process of reformation of one configuration of mass and energy into a different one. In both configurations—before and after collision—the manifest forms of matter are limited to hadron particles.

The multitude of possible hadron configurations display patterns of spin and mass that suggest that many of the shorter-lived hadron formations are higher-energy *resonances* of more stable hadron formations. These patterns are extremely similar to the resonance patterns reflected in the quantum levels of electron orbitals. On the basis of these resonance patterns as evidenced in high-energy scattering experiments, theorists have suggested that the hadrons must contain constituent elements that can exist at varied energy levels. These hypothetical elements are called *quarks*. Because hadrons do not exist except as hadrons, the quark is not experimentally discernible.[3] Quarks, therefore, are abstract inferences based on patterns, or symmetries, that are reflected in the behavior of hadrons in high-energy collision processes.

These theoretical suppositions are a result of the application of the powerful mathematics of the gauge symmetry principle to the strong interactions and have led to the formulation of the theory of quantum chromodynamics. Quantum chromodynamics is postulated as a relativistic quantum field theory, styled in terms of Yang-Mills gauge symmetry, that precisely describes the strong interactions that bind the ephemeral entities called quarks into observable entities called hadrons. The operant strong force is arbitrarily termed the *colored force* and is mediated by eight distinct *colored gluons*.

In other words, both the electroweak theory unifying electromagnetic and weak interactions and the theory of quantum chromodynamics are grounded on the principle of gauge symmetry. Accordingly, the fundamental entities believed to comprise the phenomenal universe can be classified as leptons and quarks, and all interactions between and within these elementary entities are conceived to be mediated by quanta called gluons. Each genre of interaction is conceived to be mediated by a characteristic gluon: Electromagnetic interactions are mediated by gluons called *photons*; weak interactions are mediated by three weak gluons called *intermediate bosons* W^+, W^-, *and* Z^x, and by the *Higgs gluon*; strong interactions are mediated by eight *colored gluons*; and gravitational interactions are mediated by gluons called *gravitons* and *gravitinos*.

In 1977, Howard Georgi and Sheldon Glashow published a theory that integrates the four interactions within a single symmetry that manifests only at the highest energy levels imaginable. The distinctions among the four classes of interaction are hypothesized to have evolved as lower-energy manifestations of that single, unified interaction. They are, in the words of Pagels (1982), reflections of a single, broken symmetry:

> *According to these unified theories, all the interactions we see in the present world are the asymmetrical remnant of a once perfectly symmetrical world. This symmetrical world is revealed only at very high energies, energies so high they will never be accomplished by human beings. The only time that such energies existed was in the first nanoseconds of the big bang which was the origin of the universe. (p. 263)*

Perhaps the greatest impediment to grand unified field theories involves accommodation of the gravitational interaction. Einstein was frustrated in his long ambition to unify the electromagnetic and gravitational interactions, and physicists are little closer today to solving this problem. Other substantial difficulties remain, however, even with respect to reconciling the strong interactions with the weak and electromagnetic forces. Although grand unification seems temptingly close to achievement, the remaining theoretical difficulties are not trivial.

Notes

[1]It is interesting to note that both the special and the general theories of relativity were based on operations or extrapolations from the Cartesian,

or Galileian, coordinate grid. Bohm (1983) suggests that such constancy in the conceptual framework of physics is a reflection of the very order of the phenomenal universe: "The mechanistic order is most naturally and directly expressed through the Cartesian grid. Though physics has changed radically in many ways, the Cartesian grid (with minor modification, such as the use of curvilinear coordinates) has remained the one key feature that has not changed. Evidently, it is not easy to change this, because our notions of order are pervasive, for not only do they involve our thinking but also our senses, our feelings, our intuitions, our physical movement, our relationships with other people and with society as a whole and, indeed, every phase of our lives" (p. 176).

[2]Heisenberg, at approximately the same time, developed a mathematical system of description based on matrix mechanics. Eventually, Paul Dirac (who also was the first theorist to reconcile mathematically quantum mechanics and relativity theory) demonstrated through his "transformation theory" that Heisenberg's matrix expression and Schrödinger's wave representation were essentially equivalent.

[3]In the application of quantum mechanics to hadrons—called "quantum chromodynamics"—the inaccessibility of the quark is termed "quark confinement."

8

A Conceptual Model of Mind: The Theory

*I believe that every true theorist is a kind of tamed metaphysicist,
no matter how pure a "positivist" he may fancy himself.*

Albert Einstein

Before moving beyond the Western path to knowledge, it will be instructive to review briefly the course this path has taken. The path began in chapter 2 with an investigation of the training techniques associated with high achievement in competitive athletics. In particular, this inquiry addressed the techniques for training the energy and the contractile systems of the body, which were revealed to be the principal proximate determinants of the performance parameters of endurance, strength, and power. From this analysis, it became apparent that the learning process yielding enhancements to these three performance parameters involves physiological adaptations within the functional microsystems that constitute the energy, contractile, and neuronal macrosystems. These organic adaptations are induced in response to the exercise of a limiting microsystem at or near its physiological limits. On the basis of this Physiological Model of Physical Training, it became possible to provide a meaningful interpretation of the aphorism that "practice makes perfect." This interpretation involved the extrapolation of the principle of Right Practice together with the rule of specificity of practice and the rule of intensity of practice.

Chapter 2 concluded with a recognition that the contractile and the energy macrosystems are subject to control by the neuronal macrosystem. Specifically, it was explained that a particular muscle fiber contracts in response to neuronal impulse conduction and that the intensity of the fiber's contraction is dependent on the frequency of the conduction of neuronal impulses to that fiber. By governing the selective recruitment of muscle fibers for contraction and the intensity of those contractions, the neuronal macrosystem also controls the energy macrosystem implicated in a particular motor performance. The rule of specificity of practice, therefore, contemplates the neuronal recruitment of particular muscle fibers for contraction, whereas the rule of intensity of practice contemplates neuronal control over the intensity of the contraction of the recruited fiber. Through the specificity and intensity of nerve impulse conduction, the neuronal system controls not only the performance parameters of endurance, strength, and power but also the fundamental performance parameter of coordination. Complex motor activity, in other words, can be conceived as entirely orchestrated by the neuronal system. The neuronal system therefore emerges at the conclusion of chapters 2 and 3 as the preeminent macrosystem involved in Right Practice.

From the outset, the notion of practice has been presumed to involve the concept of purpose. Purpose has been posited as the indispensable factor distinguishing practice-based learning from experience-based learning. If purpose exists within the Physiological Model of Physical Training described in chapter 2, it must be integral to the neuronal system. Early on, then, the fundamental question became whether the neuronal system harbors the element of purpose that is indispensable to Right Practice. This question was addressed in depth in chapters 4 and 5.

Purpose arises as a conceptualization within subjective awareness. On analysis, the concept of purpose was revealed to embody the two subsidiary concepts of *volition* and *attention*. The search for these states of conceptual awareness within the tissues and fluids of the body, in consonance with the Western commitment to objective empiricism, involved a rigorous empirical inquiry into the physiological processes of the neuronal system. A Physiological Model of Mind was proposed on the basis of an analysis of the electrochemical processes of neuronal conduction and the immensely complex physiological mechanisms of the brain.

This Physiological Model of Mind is based on the speculation that certain sustained, simultaneous, integrated transcortical conformations of neuronal conduction constitute the physiological substrate of subjective awareness. These unified patterns of transcortical neuronal activity have been termed hyperneuronal arcs of awareness. The hyperneuronal arc embodies an integrated network of neuronal conduction. As such, the arc's principal constituent elements are individual neurons and their junctional interfaces with other neurons.

Two primary categories of physiological processes therefore were revealed to be integral to neuronal conduction. The first category of microsystemic processes gives rise to nerve impulse conduction within the nerve cell and principally along the nerve axon. The second category produces conduction of the nerve impulse across the synaptic gap. Together, these two categories of microsystemic processes give rise to the hyperneuronal arcs of awareness. The hyperneuronal arc of awareness is therefore conceived as a spatially definite external conformation of neuronal conduction impulsing at a specific internal frequency. The external focus, or conformation, of the hyperneuronal arc is determined by the physiological processes that transpire within the microsystemic linkages of the multiple synapses joining the individual constituent neurons into an integrated, simultaneous hyperneuron. The internal focus of the hyperneuronal arc is determined by the frequency of impulse conduction sustained within that simultaneous, integrated hyperneuron.

This binary, or two-process, system of organization that gives rise to the hyperneuronal arc of awareness is the basis for informational coding within the neuronal system. The informational content of the hyperneuronal arc, in other words, is coded in terms of the external focus of the arc—that is, its specificity, consisting of the conformation of the arc within the three dimensions of brain space—and the internal focus of the arc—that is, its intensity, consisting of the frequency of impulse conduction within the arc.

The Physiological Model of Mind identifies subjective awareness as a passive, incorporeal epiphenomenon attendant on the hyperneuronal arc of awareness. Subjective awareness is understood to arise in consciousness only as conceptualization. The nature of the particular conceptualization that arises in subjective awareness, therefore, is hypothesized to be a reflection of the binary coding within the corresponding hyperneuronal arc of awareness. Concepts such as purpose, volition, and attention, for example, are understood to be reflections of the two-process coding of nerve impulse conduction.

The ultimate question became, therefore, whether these basic electrochemical microsystems comprising the binary processes of neuronal conduction are strictly mechanistic and deterministic or whether they permit the influence of original acts of mind. The attempt to answer this question took the Physiological Model of Mind deeper into the constituent microsystems, where that inquiry entered the realm of theoretical physics. Chapters 6 and 7 pursued this inquiry into these deepest domains of the phenomenal universe.

Western empiricism has marshaled its most powerful technologies and theoretical paradigms in an attempt to identify the objective laws governing the kinds of electrochemical processes involved in the microsystemic processes of neuronal conduction. Unfortunately, the best efforts of Western empiricism not only have failed to penetrate the secret recesses of such elementary processes but have proven those recesses to be inaccessible to human cognition.

The best mathematical descriptions of the fundamental processes involved in neuronal conduction are based on the theory of quantum mechanics. Specifically, the electrochemical microsystems involved in the two processes of neuronal conduction are understood to be governed principally by the laws of quantum electrodynamics that control the interactions among atomic elements. Conscious awareness, therefore, as seen through the lens of the Physiological Model of Mind, arises as a direct consequence of the highly complex interplay of positive and negative electrical charges. And this fundamentally binary system of positive and negative electrical divergencies from the dynamic equilibrium of electrical neutrality is governed by the deterministic laws of quantum electrodynamics. Yet quantum electrodynamics and quantum mechanics generally are constrained to view the quantum universe exclusively in terms of probability distributions rather than in terms of precisely measurable physical properties.

The philosophical significance of the theory of quantum mechanics has been formalized in the uncertainty principle and the principle of complementarity, which together constitute the Copenhagen interpretation of quantum mechanics. These two interpretive principles expressly recognize that the human power of cognition is fundamentally limited. Because of the inescapable relativity and imprecision of all measurement processes within the quantum domain, the elementary physical properties within that domain must remain indeterminate. Although the "laws" of quantum mechanics are rigorously mechanistic, the physical properties of the quantum realm out of which those mechanistic laws arise must remain indeterminate. It is critical to recognize, however, that the indeterminacy of the quantum realm is a function of limitations on human cognition and is not necessarily a description of or commentary on the nature of that quantum domain.

With this appreciation of the limits implicit in the Empirical Model of the Phenomenal Universe, the search for purpose—and for such other aspects of mind as volition, attention, and will—has reached an impasse. There is simply no way in which the empirical investigations of Western objectivism can reach into the secret mechanations of the quantum realm to either confirm or disprove the existence of original acts of mind as causal factors in the phenomenal universe. The mechanistic laws of quantum mechanics permit an operational analysis of the quantum domain according to which the average effects of essentially unanalyzable and unmeasurable physical systems can be known with a high degree of certainty. Yet human cognition is forever precluded from definitive empirical knowledge of the quantum domain itself. Moreover, should a subquantum level be found to exist (as hypothesized by some theorists), the limitations on cognition would merely be removed to a deeper level and would not be eliminated entirely.

The importance of this understanding of the inescapable limitations on human cognition cannot be overemphasized. It is an understanding that lies at the threshold between the objectivism of physics and the subjectivism of metaphysics and that marks the point at which acts of objective proof must give way to acts of subjective faith.

The Mind as a Deterministic Mechanism

Autonomous man is a device used to explain what we cannot explain in any other way. He has been constructed from our ignorance, and as our understanding increases, the very stuff of which he is composed vanishes. Science does not dehumanize man, it dehomunculizes him, and it must do so if it is to prevent the abolition of the human species. To man qua man we readily say good riddance. Only by dispossessing him can we turn to the real causes of human behavior. Only then can we turn from the inferred to the observed, from the miraculous to the natural, from the inaccessible to the manipulable.

B.F. Skinner

It is commonly suggested that the laws of quantum mechanics, including the laws of quantum electrodynamics, are nondeterministic. Atomic events, according to this argument, transpire randomly and therefore cannot be contained within a deterministic cosmology. On analysis, however, it becomes apparent that quantum mechanics transforms the concept of randomness into a definite physical law that must obtain in order for the statistical mechanics of quantum theory to conform with experimental evidence.

To be sure, the concept of determinism can be so limited in definition that mechanistic laws of causality and chance can be expressed outside of its contemplation. For example, Bohm (1984) suggests such a restrictive definition of determinism, limiting the concept to the "assumption that the great diversity of things that appear in all of our experience, everyday as well as scientific, can all be reduced completely and perfectly to nothing more than consequences of the operation of an absolute and final set of purely quantitative laws determining the behavior of a few kinds of basic entities or variables" (p. 37). Accordingly, Bohm distinguishes between the "determinist mechanism," best exemplified in the Marquis de Laplace's absolutist extension of Newtonian physics, and what he characterizes as the "indeterminist mechanism" of the Copenhagen interpretation of quantum mechanics.

Laplace represents one of history's most vociferous proponents of an absolute determinist mechanism. Writing in the early 19th century, this eminent French mathematician and astronomer gave unequivocal expression to a radically deterministic cosmology:

> *An intellect which at a given instant knew all the forces acting in nature, and the position of all things of which the world consists— supposing the said intellect were vast enough to subject these data to analysis—would embrace in the same formula the motions of the greatest bodies in the universe and those of the slightest atoms; nothing would be uncertain for it, and the future, like the past, would be present to its eyes.* (Capra, 1984, p. 45)

Bohm (1984) contrasts such a determinist mechanism with the indeterminist mechanism implicit in modern quantum theory (pp. 101-103). Indeterminism enters the still mechanistic processes of nature through the Heisenberg uncertainty principle, which establishes that quantum events are not cognizable in any precise and absolute sense. Within the contemplation of quantum theory, no matter how vast the perceiving intellect, fundamental physical properties must remain uncertain.

As explained in chapter 6, however, the uncertainty, or indeterminism, of quantum theory is not necessarily a statement about the physical reality itself. Rather, it is an admission of the inaccessibility of that physical reality to definitive human perception and cognition. Quantum mechanics does not mandate that quantum events occur spontaneously without antecedent causes; instead, it implies that the capacity for perception and measurement of quantum events is fundamentally limited and relative and that such events therefore must be treated, for purposes of analysis, as operationally random and indeterminate.

It is important to recognize that the laws of probability are, ultimately, deterministic. Even the concept of randomness that underpins probability theory does not hold that quantum events occur spontaneously without definite antecedent causes. Rather, events that are conceived as random within the contemplation of a physical law involve contingencies that are outside the context of the approximately autonomous physical system subject to that physical law and possess such a "complex, multifold and interconnected character" that "their average effects can, in a wide range of conditions, be treated in terms of chance fluctuations and the theory of probability" (Bohm, 1984, p. 141). Randomness, in other words, is defined operationally and possesses no absolute meaning. Simply because a single roll of a die is random to our perception, it does not follow that the specific outcome of that roll was not determined by antecedent factors remote to our perceptions. The efficacy of statistical mechanics as a mode of viewing specific physical systems to a high degree of approximation does not imply indeterminism. Instead, indeterminism, like randomness, is an operational fiction devoid of absolute meaning.

Both Laplace's determinist mechanism and the indeterminist mechanism of quantum mechanics, therefore, are contained within the broader definition of determinism that undergirds all scientific systems of cognition. For example, Bohm (1984) begins his investigation of *Causality and Chance in Modern Physics* with the following fundamental declaration:

> In nature nothing remains constant. Everything is in a perpetual state of transformation, motion, and change. However, we discover that nothing simply surges up out of nothing without having antecedents that existed before. Likewise, nothing ever disappears without a trace, in a sense that it gives rise to absolutely nothing existing at later times. This general characteristic of the world can be expressed in terms of a principle which summarizes an enormous domain of different kinds of experience and which has never yet been contradicted in any observation or experiment, scientific or otherwise; namely, everything comes from other things and gives rise to other things. (p. 1)

Bohm ends his highly sophisticated analysis of causality and chance with a similar acceptance of the ultimate determinism of the phenomenal universe:

> In fact, if it were possible to define the totality of all reciprocal relationships between things, this would enable us to define matter in the process of becoming completely. For every thing that exists, including all its characteristic properties and qualities, every event that happens, and every law relating to these events and things, is defined only through such reciprocal relationships. (p. 169)

Bohm concludes that the "qualitative infinity of nature" forever precludes human cognition of all the reciprocal relationships that "determine" the physical universe (chapter 5, sections 5-12). The fundamental presumption of determinism, however, remains as an indispensable postulate that, Bohm suggests, "is at the foundation of the possibility of our understanding nature in a rational way" (p. 1).

Ultimately, then, quantum indeterminacy simply means that it is beyond human capacity to discern the nature of the determinist mechanism that gives rise to quantum events and properties. And of course, it is also beyond human capacity to prove or to disprove that determinism prevails. The Physiological Model of Mind, grounded in the Empirical Model of the Phenomenal Universe, makes a presumption of determinism by act of faith. Virtually all Western scientific inquiry makes this same presumption by a similar act of faith. Determinism is, as Bohm emphasizes, "at the foundation of the possibility of our understanding nature in a rational way." Such fundamental aspects of rational cognition as causality and order depend on this faith in determinism.

The determinist faith of Western empiricism is grounded, then, on the single fundamental postulate that, repeating the words of Bohm, "everything comes from other things and gives rise to other things." Embodied within this postulate are all the interactions of matter and energy in space and time that constitute the cognizable phenomenal universe. "Things" constitute the matter of the physical universe, whereas energy is reflected in the causal processes of "coming from" and "giving rise to." The Physiological Model of Mind developed in chapters 4 and 5 accepts this deterministic faith and extends it to the limits of perception and cognition, limits that are explored in greater detail in chapters 6 and 7. Within this analysis, the mind is conceived as an incorporeal gestalt epiphenomenon associated with definite physical processes transpiring principally within the brain. The physical processes presumed to give rise to the experience of mind adhere entirely to the determinist faith. The experiences of mind themselves, however, lie outside that fundamental postulate of causality to which the determinist faith is anchored.

Experiences of mind, in other words, arise as neither matter nor energy. The mental awareness of a concept or idea, for example, is not a "thing" that can be delimited and measured in space and time. Nor is it a causal force or energy that can be perceived and measured through a discernible effect on some "thing." The experiences of mind, manifest in the subjective sensations of conscious awareness, are simply beyond detection, measurement, and analysis by the instruments and cognitive constructs of Western scientific empiricism.

The Physiological Model of Mind hypothesizes that experiences of conscious awareness arise only as immaterial and inconsequential epiphenomena attendant on specific organizations of matter and energy within the physical universe. Moreover, the model suggests that the particular state of awareness that arises in consciousness is strictly determined by the precise configuration of matter and energy with which it is associated. The systems of logic and rationality that underpin Western empiricism are viewed through this interpretation as mechanistic interactions among various hyperneuronal arcs corresponding to the conceptual terms of cognition. The processes of logic and rational thought, in other words, are not understood to be guided or directed by the mind but are conceived as physiologically linked episodes of hyperneuronal conduction. Just as complex cycles of biochemical reactions transpire without conscious direction, so too are the electrochemically linked physiological processes (constituting a "logical," or "rational," chain of hyperneuronal arcs) hypothesized to occur without control or direction from the mind. Subjective awareness, in the form of logic or rationality, simply follows along as a passive epiphenomenon.

Experiences of mind, therefore, are not conceived as arising spontaneously, or, in Bohm's words, as "surging up out of nothing without having antecedents that existed before." They are, in fact, conceived as caused, definitely and directly, by physical processes involving matter and energy. Yet the inclusion of mind within the determinist mechanism terminates there, for the experiences of mind are not themselves conceived to be causally determinative. Within the Physiological Model of Mind, awareness is conceived "to disappear without a trace, giving rise to absolutely nothing existing at later times." Experiences of mind, therefore, assume the peculiar role of being absolutely determined by antecedent physical processes but of determining nothing themselves. They are a mere passive and silent witness to corporeal reality.

There is, of course, no reason but sheer faith to believe that such a one-sided causal dynamic should obtain. If awareness is not cognizable in terms of matter and energy, then there is no reason why it should not arise spontaneously without antecedents. Yet if awareness is understood to be matter or energy, no matter how vaguely or tenuously, then its rise and decline must cause cognizable effects within the corporeal universe. The only way Western empiricism can conceptualize the incorporeal experience of mind is as a direct consequence of states of the corporeal physical reality. Yet such a conceptual paradigm implicitly requires that the experience of mind must itself exert causal effects on the physical reality. There is, however, no known mechanism through which such effects might be perceived or measured.

Western science confronts here a fundamental philosophical dilemma. If consciousness is conceived as entirely determined by physical processes, then it is integrated into those relationships of nature that require that it reciprocate with its own causal effects. If, on the other hand, consciousness is conceived as a subjective experience entirely separate from the physical processes of the phenomenal universe, then it remains beyond cognition in the terms of scientific empiricism.

Experiences of mind, therefore, are treated by Western science as unique phenomena that possess antecedent determinants but produce no effects. The mind is conceived as neither matter nor energy, yet it is understood to owe its existence entirely to those two aspects of the physical universe. Ultimately, then, conscious awareness is cognizable only subjectively and joins an objective reality of matter and energy in space and time by an act of faith.

Within this interpretation, the physiological processes that give rise to the experiences of mind strictly and entirely determine the very terms of cognition. The nature of the process of cognition, then, is understood to determine the substance of cognition. This is the converse of the "great truth" of *adaequatio*, which was introduced in chapter 3. Not only must the understanding of the knower be "adequate" to the thing to be known, but the thing to be known *will be* "adequate" to the understanding of the knower. Consequently, even if the phenomenal universe is definite and objective, it is cognizable only as entirely relative and observer-created. The process of cognition renders the physical reality in its own image. All of the fundamental terms of cognition employed by scientific empiricism to perceive and measure an ostensibly objective, definite physical universe—that is, matter and energy in space and time—can be understood to be direct reflections of the process of cognition. And the deterministic mechanism that orders these basic terms of reality likewise becomes simply a reflection of the process of cognition itself. The cognitive process creates the phenomenal universe.

This interpretation underscores the fundamental proposition that cognition itself is entirely and only an act of mind. Empiricism, objectivism, determinism, and subjectivism all are cognitive modalities that also are entirely and only acts of mind. Although the physiological processes that are understood to underlie cognition may determine the nature and content of cognition, they are not themselves cognition. Cognition, in other words, is not the presumed external universe. Rather, it is an internal, subjective universe of conceptual awareness. The limitations on cognition are not limitations within the external universe but are simply limitations within the internal universe of conceptual awareness.

Cognition, in other words, can be understood to be a "sense" of the mind. Just as our physical senses are limited to select fields of receptivity, so too is cognition limited. Yet the further artificial limitations imposed on cognition by the doctrines of empiricism and objectivism involve the mind limiting itself. It is precisely and only the mind's predisposition limiting understanding to the realm of empiricism and objectivism that forecloses cognition within the domain of subjectivism. In other words, by self-limiting the cognitive processes of mind to an empirical and objective frame of reference, the mind imposes limitations on the phenomenal universe. And of course the mind cannot justify such self-limitations through systems of cognition and rationality based entirely on those limitations.

If the processes of cognition are bound by the same laws of interaction as are all other physical processes, the cognitive reflection of an external universe presumably would be exactly congruent—that is, *adaequatio* would prevail. If, however, the laws of interaction controlling the processes of mind differ qualitatively from those controlling all other physical phenomena, then the reflection in cognition of the external reality presumably would be distorted. There is, of course, no way for cognition to test whether the processes of mind are qualitatively identical with the determinist mechanisms of the phenomenal universe. The presumption of reflective correspondence is an act of faith.

There are, therefore, two acts of faith that underpin scientific empiricism. The first assumes that the focus of consciousness in conceptual awareness is determined by and congruent with certain physiological processes within the brain. The Physiological Model of Mind suggests, for example, that conceptual awareness arises as a direct reflection of the external spatial conformation and the internal impulse frequency of a particular hyperneuronal arc of awareness.

The second article of faith involves the presumption that the physiological mechanisms that give rise to conceptual awareness are qualitatively identical to the deterministic mechanisms of the phenomenal universe. The hyperneuronal arc of awareness, for example, is presumed to function in conformity with the same principles of quantum electrodynamics—and, to a much lesser degree, with the principles of the gravitational, weak, and strong interactions—that control biochemical and physical processes generally.

Taken in concert, these two articles of faith make possible the presumption of scientific empiricism that cognition is an accurate representation of a definite external physical reality. And here at last, on the sands of compounded faiths, forever inaccessible to verification, rises the entire edifice of scientific knowledge.

The Escape to Freedom

> The will is a kind of causality belonging to living beings in so far as they are rational, and freedom would be this property of such causality that it can be efficient, independently on foreign causes determining it; just as physical necessity is the property that the causality of all irrational beings has of being determined to activity by the influence of foreign causes.
>
> Immanuel Kant

It is not surprising that many scientists have difficulty accepting the full implications of the Western deterministic bias. There is, of course, little problem with the application of a strict deterministic presumption to an external phenomenal universe. That presumption, in fact, is the condition precedent for scientific inquiry and rational analysis. Yet when turned against the internal realm of conceptual awareness, the presumption of determinism raises a serious and fundamental philosophical dilemma. The crux of this difficulty lies in the abrogation by a deterministic cosmology of all possibility for any thought or action to originate within an individual consciousness. A deterministic cosmology, in other words, mandates that the internal domain of conceptual awareness be understood as entirely determined by causal antecedents manifest within the external physical reality. There can be, therefore, no original, creative, or unique process of either thought or action generated from within the domain of mind. Individual free will is rendered illusory, and even the conceptual notion of an independent "self" becomes a chimera. Among the many scientists who have rebelled against such an application of the determinist presumption to the internal universe of mind are Bohm and Penfield.

Penfield rejects the absolute determinism inherent in the Physiological Model of Mind on the basis of his well-schooled but ill-defined intuition that the mind possesses an energy heretofore unknown to such sciences as biology and physics. The nature of that nondescript energy of mind and of the laws governing its interactions within the external phenomenal universe remain securely hidden from human cognition. Yet for Penfield, the faith that such an energy exists provides a potential escape from the clutches of the determinist dilemma (Penfield, 1975).

Bohm is far more definite in his rejection of a strict determinism of mind. He does not posit the existence of mysterious and unknowable causal energies that might somehow accommodate individual determinism within a more expansive determinism. Instead, Bohm (1983) distinguishes the experience of mind he characterizes as ''intelligent perception'' from all other processes of thought: "We have thus put together all the basically mechanical and conditioned responses of memory under one word or symbol, i.e., thought, and we have distinguished this from the fresh, original and unconditioned response of intelligence (or intelligent perception) in which something new may arise'' (p. 51).

Of course, Bohm cannot prove that the unconditioned response of intelligent perception is possible. Instead, he too accepts this proposition by an act of faith. And having admitted intelligent perception as an exception to the determinism of the phenomenal universe, Bohm is compelled to admit that ''the actual operation of intelligence is thus beyond the possibility of being determined or conditioned by factors that can be included in any knowable law'' (p. 52). Instead, intelligent perception is presumed to arise from ''the undefinable and unknown totality of flux'' in which the physical universe also is hypothesized to originate: ''This implies that what have commonly been called mind and matter are abstractions from the universal flux, and that both are to be regarded as different and relatively autonomous orders within the one whole movement'' (p. 53). Bohm expressly recognizes that this conceptual paradigm renders the relationship of mind to matter—that is, of the internal world of conceptual awareness to the external phenomenal universe—inaccessible to human understanding:

> If the thing and the thought about it have their ground in the one undefinable and unknown totality of flux, then the attempt to explain their relationship by supposing that the thought is in reflective correspondence with the thing has no meaning, for both thought and thing are forms abstracted from the total process. The reason why these forms are related could only be in the ground from which they arise, but there can be no way of discussing reflective correspon-

dence in this ground, because reflective correspondence implies knowledge, while the ground is beyond what can be assimilated in the content of knowledge. (p. 55)

Moreover, Bohm admits that the very existence of an "unknown and undefinable totality of flux that is the ground of all things and of the process of thought itself, as well as the movement of intelligent perception," can never be established with any certainty (p. 59). It must remain, ultimately, an article of faith.

Sir John Eccles, a Nobel Laureate in medicine and physiology, has emerged as one of the most persuasive proponents of what has come to be known as *dualist interactionism*, or the theory that nonmaterial experiences of mind can act on a material brain. Indeed, in his most recent writings, Eccles claims that a substantial body of research has demonstrated irrefutably that the incorporeal mental experience of intending a voluntary act initiates the physiological processes within the brain that eventually cause the intended act to manifest in behavior (Eccles & Robinson, 1984, pp. 162-163). Eccles, however, is no more successful than Penfield or Bohm in identifying a mechanism or agency of "liaison" between mind and brain. Instead, he too ultimately accepts dualist interactionism as an article of faith.

One of the more interesting attempts to conjure up from the cauldron of empirical evidence a potent causal agency of mind is contained in the writings of the eminent neurophysiologist Roger W. Sperry, who is one of the leaders in "split-brain" research. Sperry has formulated a sophisticated model of the mind in which consciousness is conceived "to be a dynamic emergent of brain activity, neither identical with, nor reducible to, the neural events of which it is mainly composed." Indeed, Sperry goes on to emphasize that consciousness, in this conception, is not "an epiphenomenon, inner aspect, or other passive correlate of brain processing but rather an active integral part of the cerebral process itself, exerting potent causal effects in the interplay of cerebral operations" (Sperry, 1982, p. 513). Sperry characterizes the dynamic causal power of the mind as a synergistic, emergent property:

The causal power attributed to the subjective properties is nothing mystical. It is seen to reside in the hierarchical organization of the nervous system combined with the universal power of any whole over its parts. Any system that coheres as a whole, acting, reacting, and interacting as a unit, has systemic organizational properties of the system as a whole that determine its behavior as an entity, and control thereby at the same time the course and fate of its components. The whole has properties as a system that are not reducible to the properties of the parts, and the properties at higher levels exert

causal control over those at lower levels. In the case of brain function, the conscious properties of high-order brain activity determine
the course of neural events at lower levels. (pp. 516-517)

On close scrutiny, however, Sperry's high-level emergent properties are
revealed to be subject to the same laws of mechanistic determinism that
govern the lower levels of material interaction. Although the whole may
indeed be greater than the sum of its parts, the mechanistic (and synergistic) interactions of the parts still are understood to determine the "systemic organizational properties of the system as a whole." If the properties
of the whole exert causal control over the properties of the parts, therefore, it is only because those properties of the whole have themselves
been determined by and have emerged out of the interacting properties
of the parts. Any different causal control exerted by the whole would be
"mystical" in the sense that it would be grounded on faith rather than
empirical "fact." And although Sperry appears to reject this view, even
he admits that no direct empirical proof is available either to prove or
to disprove his hypothesis (Sperry, 1982, p. 513).

In the final analysis, there is simply no interpretation of the deterministic
presumption of scientific empiricism that will accommodate self-
determination or individual will. Attempts to salvage individual will inevitably either violate the postulate of determinism or entirely segregate
an internal cosmology of mind from the deterministic cosmology pertain-
ing to an external phenomenal universe. In any case, all departures from
the strict determinism of the West are, in essence, acts of faith rather than
acts of reason or proof.

It is inevitable that the Western bias of determinism should give way,
ultimately, to a faith in self-determination. After all, within the deterministic framework, all subjective experiences of volitional or attentive
awareness must be conceived as predetermined and inconsequential
epiphenomena. All human enterprise, therefore (including writings such
as these), is rendered both inevitable and pointless. Only with the liber-
ation of causation from the strict determinism of the mechanistic models
of the universe does the possibility arise that individuals are not irrevocably and absolutely bound by external forces of control. The escape
to individual freedom requires a departure from the deterministic
presumption of scientific empiricism.

The Ascendancy of Mind

The philosophic student, however, studies the nature of matter and
discovers it to be a manifestation of Mind. Through such mentalis-
tic reflection he comes to perceive that all the different evolutionary
explanations of the universal existence are true only from the rela-

tive point of view; that all the elements, principles, energies, sub-
stances and processes out of which, it is taught, the universe has
grown are themselves mental manifestations; and that just as water
cannot be different in reality from the oxygen and hydrogen of which
it is composed, no matter how different it is from them in appear-
ance, so these images of earth, water, air and fire cannot be essen-
tially different from the Mind out of which they came. In this way
he establishes himself thoroughly in the comprehension of the ulti-
mate mentalness and hence the ultimate oneness of all things and
permits no appearance to dislodge him from this intellectual position.

Paul Brunton

It should be clear by now that there is no intrinsic reason why conceptual awareness must be understood as a passive epiphenomenon reflecting an external physical universe. Indeed, such an understanding—which might be termed "the bias of the West"—seems exactly backward. The external world, after all, arises preeminently in conceptual awareness. If creation is perceived to be ordered, conceptual awareness must exist preliminarily as the faculty of ordered perception. It is the instrument of *adaequatio*. Conceptualization, therefore, need not be understood to arise in the image of a physical reality; instead, the physical reality may be presumed to arise in the image of conceptualization. Matter and energy in space and time originate and exist as terms of conceptual awareness. The notion of an external, objective physical reality arises in conscious awareness as an extension of those terms of conceptualization from the internal realm of mind to the external phenomenal universe. Whereas scientific empiricism presumes that the internal realm of awareness mirrors an external objective reality, this opposing orientation presumes that the external phenomenal universe is a reflection of the internal realm of conceptual awareness. Either orientation must rest, ultimately, on an act of faith. The faith of the West, manifest in scientific empiricism, asserts the primacy of the external reality. The faith of the East, manifest in rigorous systems of meditative introspection, presumes the ascendancy of the internal conceptual reality.

Within the faith of the East, all creation is a projection of the experience of mind. Mind becomes the preeminent agency of creation, and the terms of cognition, including the laws of determinism, become patterns within that creation. The processes of conceptual awareness become the sole agency of creation. And the creation—that is, the external phenomenal universe—arises in the image of the instrument of creation.

This mentalist cosmology posits the focus of consciousness in awareness as the immaterial conceptual mechanism that gives rise to the entire phenomenal universe of matter and energy in space and time. The physiological and quantum mechanical models of an objective universe—as well as all objects and processes of cognitive creation—exist preeminently and possibly only as conceptualizations. This difficult understanding of the ascendancy of conceptual awareness constitutes the indispensable foundation for the Theory of Right Practice.

The "proof" of the primacy of conceptual awareness is entirely subjective. Because concepts are neither matter nor energy, they are neither discernible nor measurable in such terms. Yet conceptual awareness is itself a palpable subjective experience. The faith of the East holds simply that the experience of conceptual awareness is real and definite. The further presumption that there exists a real and definite external reality that is reflected in ordered cognition by conceptual awareness requires yet a second, subsidiary commitment of faith.

The Eastern faith in the primacy of the internal realm of conceptual awareness limits but does not violate or compromise the laws of determinism. Determinism becomes a modality of cognition rather than an exact description of a physical reality. As such, it still is conceived to govern the relationships of matter and energy in space and time. Yet once the experience of mind is accepted as the preeminent source of all such terms or modalities ordering an external physical reality, the possibility arises that conceptual awareness can incorporate alternate cognitive paradigms applicable outside the framework of a deterministic mechanism.

The decision to commit to a subjectivist frame of reference involves the acceptance of subjective awareness as the preeminent reality. Through this faith in subjective consciousness, the phenomenal universe becomes a creation of mind. The deterministic mechanism of the objective universe becomes, then, an experience of mind, and only by further inference is it anything separate from mind. The proof of the ascendancy of mind is found in the experience of mind itself. The decision to acknowledge the validity and integrity of such proof requires an act of faith. It is this faith, finally, that leads to the willpower of the mind.

The willpower of the mind, like the mind itself, must be presumed to exist outside the boundaries of an objective universe of matter and energy in space and time. Those boundaries have been revealed to manifest in the quantum domain, where science reaches the limits of empirical cognition. Beyond the quantum, the terms of cognition—matter and energy, time and space—begin to fail, and the laws of determinism are supplanted by the notion of randomness. Bohm (1983) explains the failure of cognition within the quantum domain in terms of the " 'zero-point' energies" of "wave-particle modes of excitation in any region of space." A zero-point energy is the lowest energy level cognizable within a quantum theory before the quantum equations are rendered meaningless: "Beyond this, the whole notion of space and time as we know it would fade out, into something that is at present unspecifiable" (p. 190; see also p. 176).

It is for this reason—that is, the failure of the terms of determinism within the quantum domain—that Bohm is able to hypothesize an unknown and undefinable totality of flux from which all creation, including both mind and matter, is conceived to arise. That flux is the level of existence deeper than the quantum level, deeper ultimately than the reach of cognition.

Conceptual cognition encompasses a universe of conceptual awareness that is susceptible to affirmative definition and delimitation in terms of matter and energy in space and time. It also, however, delimits without defining certain realms beyond this universe of conceptual cognition. These realms can be described in terms only of what they are not. They have no affirmative, substantive content that can be defined directly through conceptualization. They possess no affirmative properties or qualities that are conceptually cognizable. These realms are therefore only partially accessible to conceptual awareness. In a sense, conceptual cognition can only identify and define the boundaries of such realms that lie beyond the terms of matter and energy in space and time. The entry of conceptual cognition into such realms is forever barred.

Concepts arise, of course, to name these regions that lie beyond the limits of cognition. Bohm's supposition of "an unknown and undefinable totality of flux" refers to such an inaccessible region, as do such concepts as infinity, nothingness, and randomness. Yet there is no way for conceptual cognition to penetrate beyond the externally delimited frontiers of such conceptual realms.

Conceptual awareness, in other words, can delimit the boundaries of realms beyond the reach of cognition and can even attach names to such realms. Moreover, by witnessing the rise and decline of awareness at the borders of conceptual cognition, the mind can identify, in terms of conceptual awareness, modes of interaction between the bordered realms. And it is through these interactions across the borders of conceptual cognition that the faculty of individual will is conceived to operate.

This, then, is the faith that underlies the Theory of Right Practice: the faith that the mind has the capacity for self-determination. Without that capacity there could be no practice, only eternal process. Self-determination is, in short, the necessary foundation for all practice. On this fertile ground and with due respect for the forces of determinism that underpin rational thought and discourse, it is possible to construct a model of the conceptual universe that accommodates the causal force of individual will. It is only within such a conceptual paradigm that Right Practice can be found and cultivated.

A Conceptual Model of Mind

Only two possibilities exist: either one must believe in determinism and regard free will as a subjective illusion, or one must become a mystic and regard the discovery of natural laws as a meaningless

intellectual game. Metaphysicians of the old schools have proclaimed
one or the other of these doctrines, but ordinary people have always
accepted the dual nature of the world.

Max Born

In chapters 4 and 6, an elaborate determinist model of all creation was postulated, consisting of a Physiological Model of Mind grounded on an Empirical Model of the Phenomenal Universe. These inherently deterministic conceptual frameworks were posited as the source, or determinant, of the subjective and immaterial experience of conscious awareness. Now, however, the gestalt of awareness itself must become preeminent. The universe of matter and energy, time and space, brains and minds, and galaxies and quanta must become, by an act of faith, a creation of mind. An appropriate model of mind, therefore, must arise in terms of the experience of mind—in terms, that is, of the processes of conceptual awareness.

The quest for a Conceptual Model of Mind begins with a conception of *pure consciousness*, devoid of all motion and form, as the ground, or field, of all creation. Within the field of pure consciousness is the potential for all manifestations of conceptual awareness. Pure consciousness is, then, both all and nothing. It exists only in a stationary equilibrium that is at once absolutely diffuse and absolutely unified. Within the field of pure consciousness, all oppositions and relativities are reconciled in unity. Although pure consciousness has no analogue in conceptual awareness and is therefore beyond explication in any conceptual terms, it is perhaps closest in imagery to an all-encompassing field of energy that is both uniformly diffuse and absolutely without motion. And just as all things and events exist in potentiality within pure consciousness, no thing or event exists, potentially or actually, outside of the plenum of consciousness.

Awareness arises within the field of pure consciousness as a local disruption of the formless and motionless state of pure consciousness. The life force itself can be postulated as the initial impulse of disruption. Disruptions in the field of pure consciousness cause the absolute, motionless, and uniform diffusion to be disturbed. That disturbance arises as a local vibratory motion within the field of consciousness that then causes localized concentrations and correlative rarefactions of consciousness.

Such localized concentrations of consciousness, within the Conceptual Model of Mind, are conceived as focusings of consciousness. There are two aspects to the focusings of consciousness: an *internal focus* to consciousness, which represents the degree, or intensity, of concentration; and an *external focus* to consciousness, which represents the spatial localization of the concentration. The internal focus to consciousness, therefore, is a measure of the degree or intensity of disruption within the state of pure consciousness, whereas the external focus represents the extent, or spatial conformation, of the disturbance to pure consciousness. The Conceptual Model of Mind conceives of conceptual awareness as arising from the combined internal and external focuses inherent in vibratory disruptions of the state of pure consciousness.

The spatial conformation of the external focus of consciousness provides a spatial delimitation of the conceptualization that arises in awareness. The degree, or intensity, of concentration embodied in the internal focus of consciousness provides a temporal delimitation of the conceptualization that arises in awareness. Conceptual awareness arises in the field of consciousness, therefore, as a synthesis of spatial and temporal boundaries. Every episode of conceptual awareness is bounded or delimited in space and time. The internal and external focuses of consciousness determine these conceptual boundaries.

The spatial parameter to conceptual awareness implies the manifestation of concepts as matter, involving cognizable displacements of space. The temporal parameter to conceptual awareness implies the manifestation of concepts as energy, involving cognizable displacements of time. Spatial properties arise in conceptual awareness in terms of energy operations and relationships. Temporal properties arise in terms of spatial operations and relationships. Spatial properties define the cognizable states of approximately autonomous corporeality that constitute the momentary stability, or symmetry, of energy relations. Temporal properties define the processes of change inevitably and incessantly affecting cognizable formations of matter.

As with the conceptual parameters of time and space, the correlative properties of matter and energy arise in an indivisible opposition of reciprocal complementarity. The properties defining the spatial dimension of matter are measurable and therefore cognizable only in relation to standards of measurement embodied within the temporal dimension. And reciprocally, the properties defining the temporal dimension of energy are measurable and cognizable only in relation to standards of measurement embodied within the spatial dimension. Conceptual awareness arises in episodes delimited in a synthesized continuum of space and time through the reciprocal complementarity of the internal and external focuses within the field of consciousness.

Matter and energy are understood within the contemplation of the Conceptual Model of Mind to be the archetypical properties in terms of which conceptual awareness arises in consciousness. Matter is a conceptual aggregate that contains the entire universe of "things," or conceptual objects. Conceptual objects are associated with and differentiated from one another in terms of conceptual properties, which are defined through conceptual processes. Energy is a conceptual aggregate that contains the entire universe of events, or conceptual processes. Conceptual processes are associated with and differentiated from one another in terms of conceptual properties, which are defined through conceptual objects. Properties, therefore, reveal themselves to be relativistic dualities arising through the synthesis of internal and external focuses to consciousness.

This binary relativity manifests even within the genesis of conceptual awareness itself, which can be conceived to involve simultaneous differentiation from an absolute, unbroken universality and association from an absolute and universal fragmentation. Absolute differentiation and absolute association are beyond the reach of conceptual awareness. They reside merged within the formless and motionless equilibrium of pure consciousness. Yet differentiation and association arise as equal and opposing conceptual processes through which conceptual objects, properties, and processes are defined.

There is, however, a deeper level on which the duality of equal opposition must be understood. Conceptual awareness arises as the fusion of the external and internal focuses of consciousness. Local disruptions in the field of consciousness that give rise to awareness are balanced by an equal and opposing disruption in the field. And because the disruptions that arise as conceptual awareness involve concentrations, or focusings, of consciousness, the opposing disturbance must involve rarefactions, or dissipations, of consciousness. The equal oppositions to conceptual awareness exist only in the realms beyond conceptual cognition; consequently, they are not accessible to the conceptual terms of awareness. Concepts such as disorder, infinity, randomness, and nothingness name the unknowable but do not grasp or define it. Yet it is ever-present, lurking on the nonaware side of every moment.

Each moment of conceptual awareness, therefore, consists of the pulse of consciousness between a state of conceptual awareness and an equal and opposing state of nonawareness. Because the state of nonawareness lies outside of a conceptual awareness involving space and time, it is not cognizable or otherwise perceptible in awareness, and moments of awareness generally proceed as if continuous.

The pulse of consciousness in any moment is conceived as equal and opposing disruptions from a dynamic equilibrium, or center of balance. The displacements from the dynamic equilibrium define the center of balance through their equal opposition. The center of equilibrium is the balance point through which consciousness passes in its pulse from awareness to nonawareness to awareness and so on.

Heretofore, conceptualization and awareness have been treated essentially as synonymous. This is not surprising, insofar as they invariably arise conjoined and equivalent in experiences of mind. Yet conceptual awareness involves, ultimately, the union of the two distinct processes of conceptualization and awareness.

These two processes are fused into an inseparable, indistinguishable unity as they enter the moment as conceptual awareness. As latent or potential processes within the field of pure consciousness, however, they are separate and distinct. The operant distinction between awareness and conceptualization involves their differing susceptibilities to the causal forces or energies that give rise to conceptual awareness. The realm of conceptualization is controlled by the *forces of conceptual determinism*. The realm of awareness potentially is controlled by the *force of will*.

The forces of determinism are manifestations of the relationships between conceptual objects and processes. The order imposed on consciousness through conceptualization reflects patterns of interaction between matter and energy in space and time. This conceptual order constitutes the forces of determinism. It is, in essence, the same order that is the subject of description in terms of scientific empiricism.

The force of will, in contrast, potentially controls the rise of awareness within each moment of conceptual awareness. Will is neither matter nor energy, and it exists only outside of time and space. Will is an indescribable, self-actualizing causal force that originates outside the limits of conceptualization without any cognizable antecedent cause. It operates as a causal force directly and only on awareness, yet awareness is accessible to will only at the boundaries of conceptualization. Temporally, awareness is accessible to will only prior to the moment in which conceptual awareness arises. Spatially, awareness is accessible to will at the points of conceptual failure defining the limits of conceptualization.

Awareness and conceptualization are merged in the moment of conceptual awareness. Ordinarily, the forces of determinism propagate conceptualization from one moment to the next in a process of causation coextensive with conceptual awareness. The force of will modulates that deterministic causation through its effect on awareness at the temporal and spatial boundaries of conceptualization.

In the absence of will, conceptual awareness enters the moment under the control of the forces of determinism. Awareness, in such instances, conforms entirely to conceptualization as they merge in the moment of conceptual awareness. When the causal force of will acts on awareness, however, awareness enters the moment in some degree of divergence from the conceptualization generated through the forces of determinism, and awareness and conceptualization are fused in a hybrid conceptual awareness that reflects the synthesis of the forces of will and determinism.

Will therefore potentially controls the rise and decline of conceptual awareness. The force of will acts on awareness as it passes through the center of equilibrium defining the equal oppositions to the pulse of consciousness.

The Conceptual Model of Mind, therefore, can be expressed in terms of two seminal principles and their rules of operation. These principles are *the principle of conceptual awareness* and *the principle of indeterminacy*.

The principle of conceptual awareness holds that conceptual awareness is the internal and external focusing of consciousness in volitional or attentive awareness through conceptualization. Conceptual awareness is governed by four rules of operation: *the rule of relative properties, the rule of equal opposition, the rule of limits,* and *the rule of failure.*

The rule of relative properties requires that conceptual awareness arise out of the simultaneous differentiation and association of the experiential universe in terms of complementary pairs of properties that define each other through their reciprocal relationships. The archetypical properties of conceptualization are matter and energy, which are defined within the fundamental conceptual parameters of space and time.

The rule of equal opposition requires that conceptual awareness arise always in dualities of equal opposition. Each conceptual object or process contains the potential for an equal and opposing object or process. Moreover, each moment of conceptual awareness contains an equal and opposing nonmoment of nonawareness. The equal and opposing pulse of consciousness between conceptual awareness and nonawareness defines a center of dynamic equilibrium in which pure consciousness resides.

The rule of limits requires that each conceptual object within conceptual awareness possess limits in time and space. The rule of failure requires that each conceptual process within conceptual awareness also possess limits and that such limits manifest in the cessation or failure of the process. Both conceptual objects and processes are therefore strictly delimited, and those limits are defined through failure. The boundaries of each episode of conceptual awareness therefore are defined through failure.

The second pillar of the Conceptual Model of Mind is the principle of indeterminacy. This principle holds that beyond the boundaries of conceptual awareness indeterminacy reigns. The principle of indeterminacy is informed by two subsidiary rules of operation: *the rule of determinism* and *the rule of will.*

The rule of determinism governs the realm of conceptualization. This rule requires that within the limits of conceptual awareness the laws of determinism strictly govern the relationships of matter and energy in space and time. It presumes and imposes order and rationality within the realm of conceptual awareness. The chain of causality determinative of the conceptual realm, therefore, stretches from the finite conceptual past to the finite conceptual future and proceeds at all points in time and space in accordance with conceptual processes. The forces of determinism act only on and through conceptualization.

The rule of will governs the nexus between the indeterminate realm of nonawareness and the determinate realm of conceptual awareness. Will is a self-actualizing causal force that exists outside the boundaries of conceptual awareness. The force of will acts only on and through awareness.

Awareness is accessible to will only at the temporal and spatial limits of conceptualization.

Conceptual awareness, therefore, arises as one side of the living pulse of consciousness. One episode of conceptual awareness is one concept. One concept can be either relatively compounded or relatively simple. Simple concepts are compounded, and compounded concepts are simplified, through conceptual processes of association and differentiation.

One concept occupies both one unit in time and one unit in space. No more than one concept can occupy a single unit in time or a single unit in space. A moment of awareness merges the unit of time with the unit of space in conceptualization.

Conceptual awareness enters the moment as a combination of the internal and external focusings within the field of consciousness. The internal focus of consciousness involves the internal intensity, or concentration, of the focus to consciousness and reflects a conceptual delimitation within the temporal dimension. The external focus of consciousness involves the external spatial conformation of the focus of consciousness and reflects a conceptual delimitation within the spatial dimension. Through a synthesis of external and internal focuses, consciousness arises in the moment of awareness as a concept.

Concepts relate to other concepts moment to moment only through conceptual processes. A conceptualization of a pattern of relationship between conceptual objects is a conceptual process. Processes of conceptual awareness are sustained over successive moments as chains of awareness. Chains of awareness become *disciplines of mind* when they are linked through the force of will. The shortest process requires two consecutive moments of awareness, except for the discipline of conceptual awareness itself, which can arise within a single moment.

Conceptual awareness enters the moment as a synthesis of conceptualization and awareness. The forces of determinism govern the internal and external focusings of conceptualization that enter that synthesis. The force of will potentially governs the internal and external focusings of awareness that enter that synthesis. The forces of determinism and will are, therefore, merged in superposition within each moment of conceptual awareness. The force of will cannot survive into the moment of conceptual awareness. However, through the agency of awareness, subject to the control of will outside the boundaries of conceptualization, the force of will can control the moment of conceptual awareness. And by controlling the present moment of conceptual awareness, the force of will potentially controls both past and future.

This Conceptual Model of Mind accommodates and reflects the physiological and quantum mechanical models of the universe previously derived through the path of Western scientific empiricism. Yet it goes beyond the modeling of processes of matter and energy within space and time—beyond to the realm of indeterminacy where awareness becomes accessible to the force of will—beyond to the domain of Right Practice.

Right Practice is mindful practice. Mindful practice is purposeful practice. Purpose comes to the practice oriented as either volition or attention. The force of the mind, whether manifest as volition or attention, is the willpower of the mind. The forces of determinism that are controlling within the realm of conceptualization become vulnerable to the willpower of the mind at the limits of conceptual awareness in time and space. Right Practice therefore involves applying the force of will to identify and extend the limits of conceptual awareness. The training of the willpower of the mind involves a discipline of mind, and it is this discipline of mind that lies at the heart of Right Practice.

A View to the East

Actually, there are no direct and positive things that man can do to get in touch with the immeasurable, for this must be immensely beyond anything that man can grasp with his mind or accomplish with his hands or his instruments. What man can do is to give his full attention and creative energies to bring clarity and order into the totality of the field of measure. This involves, of course, not only the outward display of measure in terms of external units but also inward measure, as health of body, moderation in action, and meditation, which gives insight into the measure of thought. This latter is particularly important because, as has been seen, the illusion that the self and the world are broken into fragments originates in the kind of thought that goes beyond its proper measure and confuses its own product with the same independent reality. To end this illusion requires insight, not only into the world as a whole, but also into how the instrument of thought is working. Such insight implies an original and creative act of perception into all aspects of life, mental and physical, both through the senses and through the mind, and this is perhaps the true meaning of meditation.

David Bohm

An understanding and acceptance of the willpower of the mind as a causal agent within the phenomenal universe requires a partial abandonment of the objectivist faith of the West in favor of the subjectivist faith of the East. Many of the preceding pages are occupied in demonstrating that the Western path to knowledge can neither establish nor refute the existence of original acts of mind by means of empirical proof. The concept of practice, however, requires that the practitioner *choose* to believe in the willpower of the mind, as the alternative choice is to believe in a strict determinism that renders the concepts of both practice and choice meaningless. The choice to believe in original acts of mind implicitly involves an acceptance of the subjectivist faith of the East.

The Conceptual Model of Mind expounded in this chapter involves the grafting of the subjectivist faith of the East onto the fully developed stalk of Western knowledge. In chapter 10, that graft finally will be seen to flower into a Theory of Right Practice. The faith of the East, however, also will stand alone. Indeed, it has stood alone for millennia, and extremely sophisticated systems of mental practice have been grounded on the Eastern faith in the validity and integrity of subjective awareness.

The techniques of practice employed by the Eastern disciplines of mind, which have evolved over thousands of years, consist predominantly of meditative introspection. Introspection is understood within the Eastern traditions of mental practice to be a process through which the mind directly "senses" its own processes and operation. Viewed from the perspective of Western objectivism, introspection is no more than hypothetical, inferential reasoning based on empirical measurements of an external phenomenal universe. Whereas the introspection of the West simply involves the application of objective empirical laws of the phenomenal universe to the subjective realm of consciousness, the introspection of the East pursues the laws of consciousness directly within the mind and not within some objective external reality. The Eastern disciplines of mind, therefore, are designed to focus the mind on itself in an attempt to perceive and then to utilize the laws of consciousness within the practice.

The basic idea of turning the mind against itself in an attempt directly to perceive the laws of consciousness seems relatively straightforward. The manifold Eastern disciplines of mind, however, employ varied and highly specialized techniques designed to maximize the efficacy of such practices. Although it is axiomatic that mental practice must be mindful practice, it is far less clear precisely how mindfulness can best be infused into a particular discipline of mind.

Mindfulness, within the practice, earlier has been equated with purposefulness. The nature of the purpose associated with the Eastern disciplines of mind must remain, however, relatively abstract. Virtually all Eastern systems of meditative introspection maintain that the practice itself constitutes the purpose and that there is no cognizable purpose that is separate and distinguishable from the *process* of practice. Purpose therefore becomes, within the Eastern disciplines of mind, indistinguishable from the practice; indeed, purpose is defined operationally to be the practice. The purpose of practice, in other words, is not to achieve some ultimate goal such as mental or physical agility or even enlightenment but is simply to maximize the integrity of the practice in the present moment.

The concept of *the present moment* is absolutely integral to Eastern systems of meditation. Indeed, Right Practice cannot occur anywhere but within the present moment. The Eastern traditions of meditative introspection therefore have as their common, central theme the focusing of the mind on the present moment of subjective awareness. And consummate Right Practice ultimately requires the transformation of all of life into the present moment of conceptual awareness.

The Eastern meditative traditions employ two complementary approaches to focusing the mind within the present moment of conceptual awareness. These approaches reflect the manifestation of purpose within subjective awareness as either volition or attention. Meditative techniques that emphasize a volitional approach require the practitioner to focus the mind on some specific conceptual object or process and to maintain that focus through successive present moments of conceptual awareness. This genre of meditation is frequently referred to as concentration meditation, and it is a highly effective technique for training the volitional aspect of the willpower of the mind. Those meditative techniques that emphasize the manifestation of the willpower of the mind as attention can be categorized as insight meditation. These systems of meditative introspection require that the mind be focused in its attentive mode on the present moment of conceptual awareness. The force of will, then, turns the mind against itself in an attempt to witness the arising of conceptual awareness within the present moment.

The preceding generalizations with respect to the Eastern disciplines of mind are simplistic representations of extremely sophisticated systems of mental practice.[1] Although it is fundamentally correct to understand the essence of these systems to be the training of the mind to dwell in the present moment as either volition or attention, a multiplicity of techniques have evolved to accomplish these quintessential purposes. Not only do these techniques vary substantially in their subtlety and efficacy, but they also are integrated into elaborate systems of mental training, involving various stages and levels of practice. These systems truly represent the wisdom of the ages. And although it is the wisdom of the East, it is wisdom that has profound relevance to the design of a Theory of Right Practice that also is attuned to the substantial wisdom of the West.

It is not the thesis of this book that the way of the West should be reoriented to correspond exactly to the Eastern path to knowledge. However, the Western path to knowledge must be extended beyond its own limits and into the realm of Eastern subjectivism. And, of course, it would be sheer ignorance for Western practitioners not to find direction and guidance in the wisdom of the East on entering that subjective realm. In this regard, it is critical that the rigor and seriousness of Eastern subjective wisdom be acknowledged and appreciated. There is frequently in evidence within the West the attitude that Eastern systems of meditative introspection are frivolous and indulgent in comparison with the arduous precision and strict methodology of scientific empiricism. Without question, there are frequent instances of sloppiness and lassitude within the Eastern practices, but there is an abundance of sloppy and lazy science as well. It is, quite simply, naive to believe that the most highly refined and disciplined pursuit of introspection is any less substantial and significant than the most rigorous pursuit of scientific empiricism.

The extremely close correspondence between the conception of the mind that supports the way of the East and the Conceptual Model of Mind developed in this chapter as a consummate extension of the way of the West is, in short, not accidental. A faith in the ascendancy of the subjective experience of mind, which is a beginning point for the way of the East, is a culmination of sorts for the way of the West. The Eastern practices of mind reflect the principle of Right Practice, the principle of conceptual awareness, and the principle of indeterminacy. The Eastern techniques of meditation are designed to penetrate the veils of compound conceptualization by force of will in an attempt to turn awareness on itself in the moment of its arising. Such techniques are, in essence, entirely compatible with the Conceptual Model of Mind posited in this chapter, in which the force of will (acting through awareness) is understood to be synthesized with the forces of determinism (acting through conceptualization) within the moment of conceptual awareness.

Both the Eastern and the Western ways of knowledge conceive of the universe in terms of relative properties that arise as dualities of equal opposition. Is it so surprising, then, that there should be two opposing orientations to the path to knowledge? Indeed, it is said that the summit of universal wisdom can be approached from either side of the mountain. Ultimately, however, there is but one summit.

There is, then, no more justification for rejecting the Eastern introspective path to knowledge than there is for eschewing the Western way of scientific empiricism. They are, at heart, simply the equal and opposing aspects to the common experience of human consciousness. And just as matter and energy are understood to merge into a mysterious and transcendent unity at the boundaries of conceptualization—as, for example, in the wave-particle duality within the quantum domain—so too do the Eastern and Western ways of knowledge merge, ultimately, within a single transcendent Theory of Right Practice.

Right Practice: A Discipline of Mind

Man is asleep. He has no permanent I, no real consciousness, no will. He is a helpless puppet in the hands of outside forces. He is a being that nature has only half created. If he wishes to be complete he must complete himself.

P.D. Ouspensky

With the acceptance of the preeminence of subjective awareness, it is possible to formulate a Conceptual Model of Mind that encompasses both the deterministic mechanisms of the Physiological Model of Mind and the subjectivist faith in the willpower of the mind. This model, which is presented in this chapter, is based on certain fundamental laws of consciousness that govern subjective awareness.

The principle of conceptual awareness holds that subjective awareness arises in consciousness as conceptualization through the internal and external focusings of consciousness. Conceptualization can arise in awareness as either a conceptual object or a conceptual process. Conceptual objects encompass the universe of things, and these objects are associated with and differentiated from one another in terms of spatial properties. Conceptual processes encompass the universe of events, and these processes are associated with and differentiated from one another in terms of temporal properties.

There are four subsidiary rules that inform the principle of conceptual awareness. The rule of relative properties embodies the proposition that all conceptualization involves complementary pairs of properties that are defined only relative to each other. The fundamental conceptual parameters of awareness are the complementary properties of space and time, and the concepts of matter and energy arise as the archetypical properties within these parameters. The rule of equal opposition is a corollary to the rule of relative properties and holds that any property will be balanced by an equal and opposite complementary property. The rule of limits holds that each conceptual object that arises within subjective awareness will possess limits within the fundamental conceptual parameters of time and space. The rule of failure extends the rule of limits to conceptual processes and provides that each conceptual process, including each process of definition, is delimited by the cessation or failure of that process within the conceptual parameters of time and space.

The second basic precept within the Conceptual Model of Mind is the principle of indeterminacy. This principle postulates that indeterminacy prevails outside the boundaries of conceptual awareness. Two subsidiary rules illuminate the principle of indeterminacy. The rule of determinism holds that strict determinism is controlling within the limits of conceptual awareness. The rule of will, on the other hand, requires that the willpower of the mind be accessible to influence the forces of determinism at the boundaries of conceptual awareness.

Taken in concert, these principles and rules not only constitute a Conceptual Model of Mind but also provide a conceptual framework within which the will can become an instrument of practice. The principle of conceptual awareness, together with its subsidiary rules, holds that all conceptual objects and processes are limited in both space and time. The principle of indeterminacy, together with its subsidiary rules, provides that the forces of determinism, which are controlling within those limits in space and time, are vulnerable to the willpower of the mind at the boundaries of conceptual awareness in space and time. Conceptual awareness, therefore, must be extended to its limits in space and time if the force of will is to become accessible. This is the essence of Right Practice, and it is this essence that is explored in chapter 10.

These, then, are the principle of conceptual awareness and the principle of indeterminacy, together with the rules that govern their operation. The Theory of Right Practice evolves from the application of these principles to the principle of Right Practice.

Note

[1]Chapter 9 contains a more detailed exposition of two representative Eastern systems of mental practice: Buddhist *Vipassana* practice and Hindu yoga practice. The reader is referred to chapter 9 for an elaboration of the extremely abbreviated explanation of Eastern meditative techniques and philosophy presented here.

9

A Conceptual Model of Mind: Eastern Applications

The Buddhist does not believe in an independent or separately existing external world, into whose dynamic forces he could insert himself. The external world and his internal world are for him only two sides of the same fabric, in which the threads of all forces and of all events, of all forms of consciousness and of their objects, are woven into an inseparable net of endless, mutually conditioned relations.

Lama Angarika Govinda

Embodied within the ancient Hindu and Buddhist traditions of Asia are a variety of sophisticated systems of mental training. These practices have evolved over several thousand years, principally within ascetic and monastic orders, and reflect a system of knowledge based on subjective experience. Systems of practice range from highly stylized and ritualistic techniques to those that are relatively simple and unadorned. Religion, with its traditional theistic foundation, is frequently partnered with the mental disciplines; yet the practices can, in almost every instance, be extracted from their religious context without damage to their integrity or efficacy. They remain, however, fundamentally mystical in orientation, for the goals of practice are understood to be revealed only in the experience of the practice and are inaccessible to conceptual cognition.

The Eastern disciplines of mind begin where the Western discipline of scientific empiricism ends—that is, with a recognition that ultimate understanding is beyond the limits of conceptualization. Fundamental truths,

197

according to the Eastern systems of mental practice, can never be revealed in words or symbols (or in any other form of conceptualization) but only within and through the practice. Truth still must meet the tests of experimentation and verification, but such an inquiry is understood to be meaningful only on a purely subjective level. The ultimate laboratory is the mind, and it cannot be otherwise.

There are, of course, a multitude of distinct systems of practice within the Buddhist and Hindu religious traditions. It is beyond the scope of these writings to attempt any comprehensive review of Eastern disciplines of mind. However, an examination of two representative, but unadorned, systems of mental training—one Buddhist and the second Hindu—reveals certain essential parameters of practice that are common throughout the many particular disciplines. These parameters are fundamentally compatible with the Conceptual Model of Mind presented in chapter 8, and are extremely illuminating in terms of their techniques of application of the principle of Right Practice to the processes of conceptual awareness. They provide a brief glimpse of the Eastern path to illumination.

Buddhism

> *But he learned more from the river than Vasudeva could teach him. He learned from it continually. Above all, he learned from it how to listen with a still heart, with a waiting, open soul, without passion, without desire, without judgment, without opinions.*
>
> Herman Hesse

Many systems of mental practice are embraced by the Buddhist tradition. All of the diverse techniques, however, reflect a veneration of the sage Gautama Buddha. Buddha taught that the inherent suffering of existence could be transcended only through practices leading to a state of illumination, or enlightenment, which is itself beyond description. The Buddha's limited prescriptions for practice have evolved over the centuries into three primary traditions of practice, and within each tradition, distinct techniques of practice have proliferated. All of the traditions, however, share a commitment to some form of meditative practice.

One of the most highly evolved and powerful of the systems of meditation currently practiced and taught is *Vipassana* meditation, a discipline of mind aligned with the *Theravada* tradition of Buddhism. Even within the Vipassana school of meditation, there are a variety of distinct styles of practice. All, however, exhibit certain common characteristics that run throughout Buddhist traditions. *Living Buddhist Masters,* by Jack Kornfield, is one of the most accessible presentations of representative Vipassana meditative techniques available to Westerners (Kornfield, 1983). Most of the references in this chapter to the different Vipassana teaching masters are taken from Kornfield's work.

Vipassana systems of meditation are distinguished within Buddhist practice from *Samatha* (or concentration) practices. A full understanding of the distinction between these two practices is revealed only to those who achieve great advancement in the practices. Yet, even for the novitiate, there are obvious differences in the style and manner of practice. Samatha meditative practice involves focusing awareness with unwavering intensity on some specific conceptualization and following that conceptualization to a state of absorption. Breath is among the most frequently utilized focuses for Samatha practice. Because respiration is a constant bodily phenomenon, it is always available for abstraction as a conceptual focus to awareness. Samatha meditation, for example, might demand a focus of concentration on the intensity of breath, the duration of inhalation and exhalation, or even on the object of breath, or "breath body." The Buddha prescribed 40 alternative focuses for Samatha meditation, and these have been interpreted to include virtually anything, from mantra and visualization to infinity and nonperception. In every instance, however, the object of the focus of awareness in concentration is some conceptual object or process.

Vipassana, or insight meditation, on the other hand, attempts to direct the focus of awareness into the process of conceptualization itself rather than upon its objects. The breath is used frequently as a focus for insight meditation but in a slightly different manner from that employed by Samatha techniques. Instead of a concentrated focus of awareness on a specific conceptualization of the respiratory process, insight practice pursues a focus of awareness on the bare sensation of breath, such as the sensation of the touch of the breath as it passes the nostril tip or upper lip or the sensation of the rise and fall of the abdomen. Ultimately, Vipassana meditation involves focusing the mind on itself. It involves turning the process of perception against itself in an attempt to experience the mind in the moment of mindfulness. The essence of Vipassana meditation can best be explained through an analysis of the specific practices themselves.

Vipassana Practice

Virtually all Vipassana practices involve some degree of sitting and walking meditation. These periods are viewed as times of maximum intensity practice and can range from several hours per day to nearly the entire day and night. Potentially, and ideally, meditative practice incorporates all aspects of life. Formal meditative practice—either sitting or walking—may be a period of maximum intensity application, yet all processes of life are available as appropriate arenas for Vipassana practice.

Certain Vipassana systems place such emphasis on constant practice within the daily life that virtually all existence is elevated to the status of formal practice. Achaan Chaa, for example, a Thai Vipassana master whose techniques of practice are taught throughout northeast Thailand, combines a system of walking and sitting meditation with a meditative focus on the daily life as a balanced and reliable path to enlightenment. There is a refreshing purity of purpose and clarity of prescription in Achaan Chaa's Vipassana practice:

> *You must examine yourself. Know who you are. Know your body and mind by simply watching. In sitting, in sleeping, in eating, know your limits. Use wisdom. The practice is not to try to achieve any-thing. Just be mindful of what is. Our whole meditation is looking directly at the mind. You will see suffering, its cause and end. But you must have patience. Much patience and endurance. Gradually you will learn. . . . So, be patient. Practice morality. Live simply and be natural. Watch the mind. This is our practice. It will lead you to unselfishness. To peace.* (Kornfield, 1983, p. 48).

The many Vipassana techniques that emphasize a formal practice of sitting and walking meditation involve elaborations and refinements to the process of simply "watching the mind."

Sunlun Sayadaw

Among the most extreme and powerful systems of Vipassana meditation is the practice developed and taught by Sunlun Sayadaw and his disciples, principally in Burma (Kornfield, 1983, pp. 83-115). The serious practitioner of the Sunlun system of meditation will engage in formal sitting practice for much of the day and night. Two periods of formal sitting practice per day of 1 to 3 hours each is considered minimal.

Sunlun is perhaps the best advocate among the Vipassana masters of the need for rigorous practice. That need is based on Sunlun's disparaging assessment of the proclivities that most practitioners bring to meditative practice:

> *Unfortunately, less than perfect behavior characteristics are typical of the yogi. He is disinclined to endeavor ardently, is quick to fidget, eager to follow after lights and colors, prone to rest in areas of calm, ready to exaggerate minor successes, willing to misuse subsidiary power, liable to give himself the benefit of the doubt, afraid of un-pleasant sensation, and terrified and clumsy when the real moment of truth is offered.* (Kornfield, 1983, p. 100)

It is against this litany of lassitude and misdirection that the Sunlun method of rigorous practice is directed. The preliminary practices of the Sunlun system have two consecutive phases. Both require a solid sitting posture (with the back held straight) that can be maintained throughout the meditative practice and that forms a foundation for alert, concentrated effort rather than relaxation.

The first phase involves "strong, hard, and rapid breathing" for an extended period of time. The time element can be preset (e.g., 45 minutes to 1 hour) or vigorous breathing can be maintained until the sensations become so intense as to require that such breathing be stopped. The critical aspect of the vigorous breathing phase of the Sunlun system involves the rigorous mindfulness of the sensation of touch caused by the passage of breath past the nostril area.

Respiration is stopped on an inhalation, and the second phase of the meditation practice is entered, as the entire body of sensation becomes the focus for attention. For the duration of the meditation, the consciousness must be focused on the most pronounced sensation. The sensation must be attended by consciousness without resort to compound conceptualization. The sensation must be experienced by consciousness in its raw immediacy. Each moment must involve a new perception of sensation: "Know neither less nor more. Know it only as it is. Know whatever arises, as it arises, when it arises, in the bare fact of its arising" (Kornfield, 1983, p. 104). The mind is instructed to follow each sensation that arises and for as long as it exists. There is no control, but only bare perception.

During the initial stages of practice, the sensation of pain invariably becomes the focus of mindfulness under the Sunlun method; in fact, the express methodology is to maintain mindfulness in the direct sensation of discomfort: "Be rigorously mindful of the awareness of touch. We should be rigorously, ardently, intensively mindful. Do not rest when tired, scratch when itched, nor shift when cramped. We should keep our bodies and minds absolutely still and strive till the end. The uncomfortable truly is the norm; the comfortable will set us adrift on the current of illusion" (Kornfield, 1983, p. 101). Unpleasant sensation is regarded as an efficacious focus for mindfulness because it will attract and concentrate attention rather than permit the indolent wandering of attention. Also, however, by penetrating to the limits of unpleasant sensation—that is, by "dwelling within the sensation, watching the sensation, without thinking any thought connected with the sensation" (p. 99)—the practitioner can transcend the element of infliction that relates the sensation of discomfort to an experiencing self. Ultimately, at the limits to sensation, even the conceptualization of a self, or an "I," dissolves.

One of the principal impediments to the Sunlun system of meditation involves the tendency to permit the rigor of effort necessary to preserve bare attentiveness to itself become an object of conceptualization, thereby abrogating attentiveness to sensation in the moment of concentrated effort. Sunlun therefore suggests that effort gradually be increased only after the attention has been firmly affixed to a sensation, by those increments compatible with maintenance of attentiveness, and never so much that effort becomes the object of attention itself.

The essence of the Sunlun system is deceptively simple: "Be rigorously mindful of the sensation of touch." Through the practice, the meditator pursues sensation toward the bare act of perception. At that rudimentary level of perception, not compounded through processes of conceptualization, "the meditator's mind becomes cleansed, purged, firm, and serviceable. . . . With cleansed, purged, firm, and serviceable mind he contemplates consciousness in consciousness" (Kornfield, 1983, p. 109).

Mahasi Sayadaw

The essence of Vipassana practice involves this attempt to focus consciousness on itself. The rigorous pursuit of sensation into the moment of its arising is a common technique to achieve this aim. The system of Vipassana meditation prescribed by master Mahasi Sayadaw, for example, requires the partnering of each sensation, as it arises, or in the moment of its arising, with a basic conceptualization of that sensation (Kornfield, 1983, pp. 51-81). Specifically, the technique of meditation taught by Mahasi involves a conceptual notation of each awareness of body or mind as it arises in consciousness. Mahasi requires extreme specificity in defining the sensation in conceptual terms. In fact, this partnering of awareness and conceptualization is the primary initial technique of his meditative system. By defining sensation with increasingly greater specificity, the consciousness is thrust into the sensation and penetrates ever closer to the bare awareness. So, for example, even within the most basic of Mahasi's meditative exercises, there is an attempt not only to distinguish and recognize each discrete act of body,[1] but to distinguish and note even the mental process of intention that precedes each volitional movement.

Formal practice under this system consists of approximately 16 hours per day of sitting and walking meditation. Clearly, it is intensive in its commitment to subject all acts of body and mind to the focus of awareness. As in virtually all systems of Vipassana meditation, the awareness of breath (in this case through the sensation of the rise and fall of the abdomen) is identified as the proper repository for awareness when it is not directed elsewhere.

This process of thrusting the consciousness after an increasingly specific awareness of sensation is reflected in Mahasi's explanation that "each act of knowing has the nature of 'going toward an object.'" The object (i.e., a specific conceptualization) and the act of knowing (i.e., the experience of awareness) are partnered; that is, they exhibit a "pairwise occurrence" (Kornfield, 1983, p. 67). After much intensive practice, the meditator's insight will become clear and precise: "He will come to perceive more distinctly the arising and disappearing of the bodily and mental processes. He will come to know that each object arises at one place and on that very place it disappears. He will know that the previous occurrence is one thing and the succeeding occurrence is another" (p. 74). This system of meditation involves an attempt to push consciousness to the limits of the two fundamental parameters of conceptualization: space and time. When Mahasi declares that "each object arises at one place and on that very place it disappears," he is isolating the spatial dimension of conceptualization for the focus of consciousness. When he discusses the awareness of an increasingly rapid succession of birth and decay for all objects, he is isolating the temporal dimension for the focus of consciousness. By pressing each object to the limits of the conceptual process, the meditator turns the focus of consciousness back against the processes of consciousness.

This emphasis on the transience of all states of mind and matter is cardinal to Vipassana practice. Samatha meditation, on the other hand, involves "concentration, whereby the individual is constantly conscious of one object, and this concentration is directed along a single channel of one-pointedness until a serene tranquility is reached" (Kornfield, 1983, p. 134). Samatha meditation therefore fosters an illusion of permanence and tranquility, whereas Vipassana meditation cultivates an awareness of the impermanent and transitory nature of mental states and matter. Even the self—the "I"—when perceived through the powerful lens of insight meditation becomes simply an illusory continuity masking the extremely rapid rise and decline of mental states and matter.

Mogok Sayadaw

The pursuit of awareness into the moment of perception reveals that awareness never remains the same for two consecutive moments. By the time awareness occupies a moment in perception, that moment has passed. Perception of perception requires at least two moments of awareness. The moment of perception can itself be perceived only in the subsequent moment, and by then it exists only in conceptualization. In presenting his system of meditation on consciousness, Vipassana master Mogok Sayadaw describes this realization, which comes to the meditator with practice:

> The life span of consciousness is momentary. When one moment of consciousness is observed it will be found that that consciousness has already vanished because the life span of any aggregate is only momentary. By the time it is observed it has passed away. One consciousness arises after another which has already vanished. Therefore, when contemplating, the yogi discovers that the consciousness upon which he contemplates has already perished. (Kornfield, 1983, p. 224; see also pp. 209-232)

The teachings of Mogok also include a Vipassana practice involving a meditation on feeling. The crux of Mogok's system of meditation on feeling is the pursuit of feeling to its point of origin in time and space. Feeling must be experienced in its time and place of arising, in the moment of its arising. The objective is to establish a rhythm of feeling and insight—of sensation and conceptualization—in successive moments of awareness such that conceptualization is pressed ever closer to the limits of cognition. And here, on the border of conceptual cognition, there is no time for awareness to conjure up the many layers of abstraction that constitute defilements, as, for example, aversion, craving, attachment, and self. Instead, Mogok's meditation on feeling involves the focus of awareness on the rise and fall of each moment of feeling, just as his meditation on consciousness requires the focus of awareness on the rise and decline of each moment of consciousness:

> *It should be cognized and seen with insight that each feeling is transient, impermanent, and never remains the same for two consecutive moments. . . . It is generally and wrongly believed that feeling is one long continuous experience, but with mindfulness and concentration the yogi will see all feeling as arising and ceasing moment to moment.''* (Kornfield, 1983, p. 229)

Common Themes in Vipassana Practice

At base, then, virtually all of the systems of Vipassana meditation demonstrate the same essential aim: to press the focus of awareness as far as possible into the process of perception. Not surprisingly, such a practice leads always to the same realization: that matter and mental states (i.e., sensation and consciousness) are ultimately momentary, transient, and discontinuous. These same words describe, within the confines of language, the conceptual limits of time and space. Awareness, through a focus in attention, is able to press through the illusion of continuity and permanence to a realization that the terms of cognition are themselves limited. And so too, therefore, is the process of perception limited.

Achaan Jumnien, a young Thai Vipassana master who teaches a meditation system that draws on virtually all of the techniques described so far, has characterized the realization that comes with practiced mindfulness:

> *The mind becomes so clear and balanced that whatever arises is seen and left untouched with no interference. One ceases to focus on any particular content and all is seen as simply mind and matter, an empty process arising and passing away of its own, or seen as just vibrations or energy, empty experience. It is out of a perfect balance of mind with no reactions that we find true liberation, beyond suffering, beyond self.* (Kornfield, 1983; p. 279)

Initially, most Vipassana practices employ a focus of awareness on sensation. Ultimately, however, all Vipassana practices involve a focus of awareness on the process of awareness itself. The process is beyond conceptualization, for it is prior to conceptualization. Vipassana practice trains the will to bring attention to the moment. In the process, awareness is turned squarely on itself. It cannot perceive itself in terms of time and space, for it is beyond the limits of both, prior to both. It can perceive itself only within the practice of a discipline of mind.

Samatha meditation, seen in this light, involves training the will to bring volition to the moment. Samatha practices focus awareness within a chain of volition that sustains a single conceptualization across consecutive moments of awareness. That single conceptualization must be a conceptual object, however compounded or simple. It is sustained, moment to moment, in volition. When a particular state of conceptual awareness is sustained through volition across multiple successive moments of awareness, the state is called *absorption*. Absorption is the goal of Samatha meditation. Volition is trained to come to the moment, then, as a conceptualization. For this reason, it is difficult to breach the limits of conceptualization through volition. The Samatha meditation techniques that do attempt to turn volition against the limits of conceptualization cast volition as some "nonconceptualization" such as infinity or probability, absolute differentiation or absolute association, or the present moment.

Vipassana meditation, however, favors the receptive, centripetal mode of attention above the projective, centrifugal mode of volition. The process of conceptualization itself is the ultimate discipline, and it is the only conceptual process that can be contained within a single moment of awareness. Through the Right Practice of Vipassana meditation, the practitioner focuses awareness as attention on its own entry into the moment in each successive present moment of conceptual awareness. Attention witnesses awareness arise within the moment. Proper insight meditation involves an unbroken chain of such moments of attention to awareness.

There is, within Vipassana practice (and within Buddhism generally) a strong implication of determinism. In the words of U Ba Khin, a meditation master who also was a major figure in Burmese government for many years, the meditator "emerges out of meditation with a new outlook, alive to the fact that whatever happens in this universe is subject to the fundamental laws of cause and effect. He knows with his inward eye the illusory nature of the separate self" (Kornfield, 1983, p. 248).

This deterministic bias must be understood only as a prescription for formal practice: Vipassana meditation places the attention in the moment, where there is no room in time and space for any conceptual process implying causality, including the continuity and coherency of self. So long as any conceptual sense of self survives during practice, the practice is imperfect.

Practice would not be practice, however, if the deterministic model prevailed absolutely. It would be process only, and there could be no discipline of mind. Taken to its limit, determinism involves the supposition that there can be no acts of mind or matter that originate within any individual, distinguishable organization of mind or matter. In other words, all acts or behavior of all objects, animate or inanimate, would be strictly predetermined. Such an explicit statement of the determinist perspective is rare in the Vipassana tradition. It is difficult to sustain a practice that is conceived as predetermined.

This apparent paradox involved in striving rigorously with selfless detachment—of practicing without practicing—strikes to the heart of the Buddhist tradition. Buddha's last words before his entry into *parinirvana* were, "Decay and impermanence is inherent in all compound things. Work out your own salvation with diligence" (Kornfield, 1983, p. 249). There is, in this statement (and in many other statements by Buddha), a very strong implication of individual will. Were all aspects of this universe strictly predetermined, an exhortation to "work out your own salvation with diligence" would be meaningless. One would work out one's salvation according to the dictates of determinism.

Without question, the karmic wheel turns heavily throughout Buddhist doctrine; yet there is just as clearly an implicit promise of individual will. It is, in essence, the will that is trained through the practices. Yet when the will finally is able to sustain a focus of attention in the moment, there simultaneously cannot be any perceiving self. And without a self, there can be no individual will. This apparent paradox involved in training the will to perceive its own illusoriness is resolved only by the realization that the will exists exclusively outside the boundaries of conceptualization. Will is a causal force accessible prior to each present moment but is absolutely inaccessible within conceptualizations that arise through a succession of such present moments.

With extremely few exceptions, the practice is never completed. It is a self that practices, and that self dwells in the conceptualization of causality and continuity of time and space. The practice is, ultimately, a way of life, and the end of practice comes only at the end of life. Vipassana practice is a process and not a product. It is a discipline of mind:

> [The practice] itself is the goal because each moment that you are mindful, fully in the present, freed from greed, hatred, and delusion, is a moment of liberation as well as a step toward final liberation. Spiritual practice becomes, at a minimum, a lifelong task; unless one is totally liberated and fully enlightened, there's always more to be done. (Kornfield, 1983, p. 300)

Hinduism

The practice of Yoga induces a primary sense of measure and proportion. Reduced to our own body, our first instrument, we learn to play it, drawing from it maximum resonance and harmony. With unflagging patience we refine and animate every cell as we return daily to the attack, unlocking and liberating capacities otherwise condemned to frustration and death. Each unfulfilled area of tissue and nerve, of brain and lung, is a challenge to our will and integrity, or otherwise a source of frustration and death.

Yehudi Menuhin

A different perspective on meditative practice is reflected in the predominantly Hindu traditions of yoga. Although there are as many different systems of yoga throughout the Hindu world and beyond as there are differing traditions of Buddhism, and although these systems have proliferated in various incarnations throughout the West, the fundamental practices of yoga are relatively constant. These fundamental practices were subject to one of their earliest and most definitive codifications in the *Yoga Sutras* of Patañjāli (Patañjāli, 1953).

Yoga, like Vipassana practice, specifies that its teachings will be revealed only through and within the practice. Theoretical writings abound with respect to yoga, of course, but the essence of the teachings cannot be found elsewhere than within the practices themselves. Among the most thorough and precise expositions of yoga practice available to Westerners are the works by master B.K.S. Iyengar, on hatha yoga and prāṇāyāma: *Light on Yoga: Yoga Dīpka (1977)* and *Light on Prāṇāyāma: The Yogic Art of Breathing (1981)*. Iyengar's treatises provide the principal basis for the exposition of yoga practice contained in this chapter.

For most Westerners, the practice of yoga is conceived as a set of postures involving varying degrees of bodily contortion and perhaps as sitting meditation. In fact, however, yoga is an extremely sophisticated system for focusing awareness:

The word 'yoga' is derived from the Sanskrit root 'yug' which means to bind, join, attach and yoke, to direct and concentrate the attention in order to use it for meditation. Yoga . . . is the art which brings an incoherent and scattered mind to a reflective and coherent state. It is the communion of the human soul with Divinity. (Iyengar, 1981, p. 4)

The Hindu religion, out of which the traditions of yoga have evolved, is fundamentally polytheistic. Iyengar does not divorce his practice or teaching of yoga from the strong religious roots to which it historically is tied. References to some abstract divinity or to specific chosen deities are common within Iyengar's texts, as are references to theological mythology. Yet the practices of yoga are preeminently and essentially a discipline of the mind rather than a body of religious ritual. The invitation to yoga contained in R.R. Diwakar's foreword to Iyengar's *Light on Prāṇāyāma*, distinguishes this discipline from the religious context in which it was sired:

> *Here I would assert that Yoga is not a part of any religion with a theology and ritualism. It has no hierarchy. It is a cultural and spiritual discipline open to all mankind without any distinction of caste, creed, color, race, sex or age. Perhaps the only essential qualification is a belief in the potentialities of one's own consciousness and an aspiration to reach its summit by following the laws of consciousness itself.* (Iyengar, 1981, p. xviii)

The essence of yoga, in other words, is the application of the laws of consciousness in pursuing consciousness to its highest levels. Yoga, then, is a system for training consciousness—that is, a discipline of mind.

The laws of consciousness that yoga embodies do not vary across cultures or among individuals. They are everywhere and always the same. Right Practice reflects an understanding and exploitation of these laws, whether the practice be yoga, Vipassana meditation, mathematics, athletics, or any other discipline. Not surprisingly, then, yoga is founded on the principle of Right Practice. As Iyengar (1977) admonishes the aspiring yogi, "Constant practice alone is the secret of success" (p. 30).

The Eight Limbs of Yoga

The specific practices of yoga are expounded by Patañjāli to include eight "limbs," or stages, which represent levels of practice in the pursuit of an ultimate state of enlightenment. They are not necessarily practiced sequentially or exclusively of one another; however, each of the eight levels provides a basis from which the next proceeds.

Yama and Niyama

Insofar as these Eastern disciplines are profoundly subjective in approach, they characteristically place great importance on the cleansing and purification of the practitioner's body and mind. The techniques of purification designed to sensitize and fortify the subjective consciousness generally are regarded as indispensable preliminaries to the actual practices of introspection. In Buddhist Vipassana practice, for example, strict and frequently elaborate rules of conduct usually circumscribe the various formal practices. Similarly, morality and purification are the subjects of the first two limbs of yogic practice: *Yama* and *Niyama*.

Yama consists of "universal moral commandments or ethical principles," such as truthfulness, nonviolence, noncovetousness, continence, and nontheft (Iyengar, 1977, p. 21; 1981; pp. 5-7). Niyama consists of rules of conduct for self-purification, such as purity, contentment, austerity, self-study, and dedication to the divine (see Iyengar, 1977, pp. 36-40; 1981, p. 7). All of these specific components of Yama and Niyama are purposeful and complex, and they have implications that transcend the ordinary meanings of the words. They constitute a system of conduct that is designed to bring every act of body, speech, and mind into the realm of Right Practice. Through Nama and Niyama, the body and mind are prepared for the formal practices that comprise the heart of yoga.

Āsana

The third limb of yoga is really the beginning of the formal practices. Patañjāli names this stage Āsana, and it constitutes that system of practice commonly known as hatha yoga. Superficially, the practice of Āsana is a discipline of the body. It involves an extremely sophisticated and comprehensive system of bodily postures designed to exercise and stimulate every aspect of the physical and subtle, or immaterial, body:

> Āsanas have evolved over the centuries so as to exercise every muscle, nerve, and gland in the body. They secure a fine physique which is strong and elastic without being muscle-bound, and they keep the body free from disease. They reduce fatigue and soothe the nerves. But their real importance lies in the way they train and discipline the mind. (Iyengar, 1977, p. 40)

There is no simple or concise way to describe the system of yogic postures that comprises the Āsana limb of yoga. Iyengar's *Light on Yoga* contains a detailed description of over 200 distinct āsanas, each with its own particular purpose and technique. Selected regimens of āsanas provide rigorous preliminary practices intended to discipline the body and mind in preparation for the higher practices of yoga.

Prāṇāyāma

The fourth level of yogic practice is termed Prāṇāyāma and consists of the discipline of the breath. In fact, it is within the practice of Prāṇāyāma—together with the practices of the fifth limb of yoga, Pratyāhāra—that the discipline of the breath reaches a culmination.

The yogic concept of breath, however, is not understood in only its narrow aspect as that process by which the lungs are filled and emptied. Instead, breath is subsumed within the broader concept of prāna, which is understood to include "breath, respiration, life, vitality, wind, energy, or strength" (Iyengar, 1977, p. 43). Iyengar (1981) presents a definition of this expansive concept of prāna:

> It is as difficult to explain *Prāna* as it is to explain God. Prāna is the
> energy permeating the universe at all levels. It is physical, mental,
> intellectual, sexual, spiritual and cosmic energy. All vibrating ener-
> gies are prāna. All physical energies such as heat, light, gravity, mag-
> netism and electricity are also prāna. It is the hidden or potential
> energy in all beings, released to the fullest extent in times of danger.
> It is the prime mover of all activity. It is energy which creates, pro-
> tects and destroys. Vigor, power, vitality, life and spirit are all forms
> of prāna. (p. 12)

Although the breath of respiration is but one of the manifestations of prāna
within the body, it is the most accessible to consciousness. It is this accessibility that is used by the yogi as a focus for the practice of Prāṇāyāma.
Superficially, the practice of Prāṇāyāma involves the conscious control
of the depth and rhythm of respiration. There are four parts to the respiratory cycle within the contemplation of Prāṇāyāma: inhalation, or *pūraka*;
exhalation, or *rechaka*; and retention, after full inhalation as *anatara kumbhaka* or after full exhalation as *bāhya kumbhaka*. With each inhalation, the
body absorbs the fundamental energy of prāna. During retention that
prānic energy is circulated throughout the body. With exhalation, the body
purges toxins and vitiated air:

> Inhalation is the act of receiving the primeval energy in the form of
> breath, and retention is when the breath is held in order to savour
> that energy. In exhalation all thoughts and emotions are emptied
> with breath: then while the lungs are empty, one surrenders the in-
> dividual energy, 'I', to the primeval energy, the Ātmā. (Iyengar, 1981,
> p. 10)

There is far more to Prāṇāyāma practice, however, than control of the
depth, intensity, and rhythm of respiration. Prāṇāyāma is actually a system of complex manipulations of respiratory function designed to direct
the circulation of prāna through a vast internal network of bodily channels called *nāḍis*.

Prāṇāyāma practice cannot be understood without a basic comprehension of the yogic conception of this subtle or causal body. The nāḍis form
the energy conduction system for the body, through which the energy
of prāna flows. Ancient yogic texts number the nāḍis at 350,000 or more,
and they are both physically discernible and subtle, or immaterial, in con-
stitution. The nāḍis are not only the "arteries, veins, capillaries, bron-
chioles and so on" but also the "channels for cosmic, vital, seminal and
other energies as well as for sensations, consciousness and spiritual aura"
(Iyengar, 1981, p. 32).

Of the approximately 14 major nāḍis, three are preeminent: the *suṣumṇā*,
the *iḍā*, and the *pingalā*. The suṣumṇā is the central and dominant of these

three principal nāḍīs. It runs through the center of the spine and represents fire. The iḍā and the pingalā nāḍīs run along the right and left sides of the suṣumṇā, also in the vicinity of the spinal cord. The iḍā, which terminates in the left nostril receives the energy of the moon. The pingalā terminates in the right nostril and receives the energy of the sun. The suṣumṇā, iḍā, and pingalā have 11 significant junctions, or plexuses, between the base of the spine and the top of the head. These nāḍi junctions, of which seven are paramount, manifest as radiating energy centers and are called *chakras*. Although the chakras may have some physically discernible aspects, they are primarily manifestations of the subtle body, lacking in materiality.

The prānic energy that is conducted through the nāḍīs also is beyond measurement in physical terms. It is called *bindu*, "literally a point having no parts and no magnitude" (Iyengar, 1981, p. 36). Bindu enters the nāḍīs principally, though not exclusively, through inhalation. Prāṇāyāma employs highly evolved respiratory techniques—specifically, āsanas (postures), mudrās (seals), prāṇāyāmas (regulation of depth, intensity, and rhythm of respiration), and bandhas (locks)—to concentrate and direct the prānic energy of bindu within the pervasive network of nāḍīs.

The culmination of this practice is conceptualized in certain systems of Prāṇāyāma to consist of the awakening of the *Kuṇḍalinī* power, located at the base of the spine, and the raising and uniting of this tremendous power with the *sahasrāra chakra* (or supreme soul) at the top of the head. Iyengar (1981) explains:

> According to the Tantric texts, the object of prāṇāyāma is to arouse the latent power (sakti) called kuṇḍalini, the divine cosmic energy in our bodies, lying at the base of the spinal column in the mūlādhāra chakra, the nervous plexus situated in the pelvis above the anus at the root of the spine. This energy has to be aroused and made to ascend through the suṣumṇā from the mūlādhāra chakra to the thousand-petaled lotus (sahasrāra) in the head, the net-work of nerves in the brain. After piercing the intervening chakras, it finally unites with the Supreme Soul. This is an allegorical way of describing the tremendous seminal vitality which is obtained by the practice of uddiyana, mula bandhas and self-restraint. It is a symbolic way of describing the sublimation of sexual energy. (p. 37)

There is no question that Prāṇāyāma practices, such as the techniques employed in Kuṇḍalinī yoga, are extremely powerful. The literature abounds in strong cautions against uninformed, unsupervised practice. Yet that same power, when utilized with skill and knowledge, can be an extremely potent force in focusing awareness. The concentration and direction of prānic energy through practices of Prāṇāyāma puts the infinite power of prāna into the service of awareness.

Pratyāhāra

It is through the practices of Pratyāhāra, designated by Patañjāli as the fifth limb of yoga, that Prāṇāyāma is turned against the domination of awareness by the senses. Pratyāhāra involves techniques of rhythmic breathing coupled with a system of conceptualization that "quiets the senses and draws them inwards" (Iyengar, 1981, p. 10). It is through these practices that awareness escapes from the tyranny and dominion of the senses.

These first five limbs of yoga create a body and mind that are highly disciplined. Yogic practice culminates, then, within the sixth, seventh, and eighth limbs of yoga, in which this highly disciplined mind is turned on itself in meditative practice.

Dhāraṇā

The sixth limb of yoga is termed *Dhāraṇā*, which closely resembles the Samatha meditation practices within the Buddhist traditions. Through the practice of Dhāraṇā, the awareness is stilled and focused on a single object, leading ultimately to a state of "complete absorption" (Iyengar, 1977, p. 48). The yogic tradition categorizes mental states according to five classifications, ranging from a consciousness that is extremely scattered and diffuse to one that is highly resolved and concentrated. Dhāraṇā involves the systematic cultivation of this highest state of concentration, or focus, of consciousness.

Dhyāna

The practice of Dhāraṇā, when pursued to the level of absorption and maintained, merges into *Dhyāna*, the seventh limb of yoga.

> Dhyāna means absorption. It is the art of self-study, reflection, keen observation, or the search for the Infinite within. It is the observation of the physical processes of the body, study of the mental states and profound contemplation. It means looking inwards to one's innermost being. Dhyāna is the discovery of Self. (Iyengar, 1981, p. 223)

The state of absorption to which Iyengar refers in this passage is strikingly similar to the absorptive states designated in the Buddhist traditions of meditation, involving a merging of the knower and the object known in the process of knowing: "Dhyāna is the full integration of the contemplator, the act of contemplation and the object contemplated upon becoming one" (Iyengar, 1981, p. 223). Within the Vipassana tradition of meditation, such absorptive states are considered the culmination of concentration, or Samatha, practice. However, when the techniques of contemplation embodied in Dhyāna practice are turned against the process of consciousness itself, the practice becomes virtually indistinguishable from insight, or Vipassana, meditation. Dhyāna practice, like Vipassana practice, climaxes with the union of the object of contemplation, the process of contemplation, and the contemplator in the moment of contemplation.

At the highest levels of attainment, Dhāraṇā and Dhyāna practices, like Samatha and Vipassana practices, are not easily distinguishable. Ultimately, however, the operant distinction appears to turn on whether the practice involves a focus of awareness in projection or in reception. Dhāraṇā practice, in these terms, is projective, or volitional. Dhyāna practice, on the other hand, is receptive, or attentive. Although Iyengar does not expressly recognize this division, it is implicit in his description of the distinction between the state of stillness and the state of silence:

> [The state of stillness] is achieved by controlled discipline of the body, the senses and the mind. It should not, however, be mistaken for silence. In stillness there is rigidity due to force of will. Here the attention is focused to keep the consciousness (chitta) still (dhāraṇā), whereas in silence that attention is expanded and released (dhyāna) and the will is submerged in the Ātmā. This subtle distinction between stillness and silence can be known only by experience. (Iyengar, 1981, pp. 232-233)

This quotation is extremely revealing. In stating that the "will is submerged in the Ātmā" through the expansion of consciousness in Dhyāna practice, Iyengar suggests that consciousness, when focused in an entirely receptive mode, can receive and become absorbed in the bare processes of consciousness. This is, essentially, the goal of Vipassana practice as well.

Samādhi

This final level of absorption within the moment of awareness is, of course, beyond the cognizance of any system of conceptualization based in time and space. It is, as virtually all masters of virtually all traditions state, inexpressible in language or symbol, and can be realized only through experience in the practice.

It is this ultimate state of nonconceptual illumination that constitutes the eighth and final limb of yoga: *Samādhi*. This highest level of yogic practice, which transcends cognitive awareness, is described by Iyengar (1981) as "the Eternal Now, beyond space and time" (p. 233).

Note

[1]For example, Mahasi admonishes, "You must attend to the contemplation of every detail in the action of eating: When you look at the food, looking, seeing. When you arrange the food, arranging. When you bring the food to mouth, bringing. When you bend the neck forward, bending. When the food touches the mouth, touching. When placing the food in the mouth, placing. When the mouth closes, closing. When withdrawing the hand, withdrawing. Should the hand touch the plate, touching. When straightening the neck, straightening. When in the act of chewing, chewing. When you are aware of the taste, tasting. When swallowing the food, swallowing. Should, while swallowing, the food be felt touching the sides of the gullet, touching." (Kornfield, 1983, p. 63)

10

A Discipline of Mind: The Theory

Focus your attention on the link between you and your death, without remorse or sadness or worrying. Focus your attention on the fact that you don't have time and let your acts flow accordingly. Let each of your acts be your last battle on earth. Only under those conditions will your acts have their rightful power. Otherwise they will be, for as long as you live, the acts of a timid man.

Don Juan, Carlos Castaneda

Finally, this book returns to the notion that practice makes perfect. Now, however, this fundamental maxim can be viewed through the powerful lens of the Conceptual Model of Mind. In this chapter, the paths of the West and the East will be merged into a single Theory of Right Practice premised on a discipline of mind. This system of learning involves the application of the principle of Right Practice enunciated in chapter 2 to the principle of conceptual awareness and the principle of indeterminacy enunciated in chapter 8. Ultimately, the discipline of mind involves the training of the willpower of the mind, and Right Practice involves the purposeful use of the willpower of the mind.

The Theory of Right Practice is grounded entirely on the willpower of the mind. Process becomes practice only through the operation of the individual will. Will is the exception to the absolute determinism of the phenomenal universe of matter and energy in space and time. As such, will becomes the agency for original acts of mind and body, bringing purpose and meaning to an existence otherwise doomed to the utter insignificance of strict determinism.

The forces of determinism, as described in chapter 8, will manifest in conceptual awareness even in the absence of any exercise of will. This, in fact, is the normal condition of waking consciousness for most individuals. The common flow of human enterprise is substantially devoid of will. To be sure, the subjective experience of conceptual awareness frequently attends such activities, but it is an awareness untouched, or barely touched, by will. Even unwilled acts of body and mind can, of course, engage human consciousness fully, even passionately. Indeed, both the forces of determinism and the force of will play on the same field of pure consciousness. Yet without the exercise of will, conceptual awareness is strictly dictated by the forces of determinism. It is, therefore, the uncommon episode of conceptual awareness that escapes the fetters of strict determinism.

For most individuals, then, daily life is carried from one moment of conceptual awareness to the next on the currents of determinism. Whatever subjective sense of control or free will such an individual might enjoy is largely illusory. Although awake to conceptual awareness, the individual remains asleep to the uniquely human possibilities of individual will. It is, in essence, a life of mere process, undistinguished by practice.

In the absence of will, the forces of determinism are propagated from one moment to the next unmolested by any extraneous causal agency. The forces of determinism are themselves the operant manifestation of the order of the conceptual universe, involving patterns of relationship between matter and energy in time and space. Undisturbed by the force of will, the forces of determinism will dictate the external and internal focuses to conceptualization—that is, its spatial and temporal dimensions—which will be mirrored within the moment by the external and internal focuses of awareness. In the absence of will, consequently, the forces of determinism indirectly control the focuses of awareness. The state of conceptual awareness that arises within the moment is entirely defined in such instances by the forces of conceptual determinism.

The escape from the clutches of determinism must be made through the force of will. Will is, ultimately, beyond direct definition. It arises as an immaterial causal force beyond the boundaries of conceptualizations involving time and space. It is discernible as neither matter nor energy. Yet will is the sole and indispensable instrument of practice.

The force of will operates exclusively on awareness, and awareness arises in consciousness only conjoined with conceptualization as conceptual awareness. The force of will cannot enter or directly act on the realm of conceptualization. By control of awareness, however, will is able indirectly to determine the state of conceptual awareness that arises within the present moment. Awareness is accessible to will only at the center of dynamic equilibrium that defines the equal oppositions to the pulse of consciousness. As consciousness passes through that center of equilibrium in its pulse from nonawareness to awareness, the force of will potentially controls the external and internal focuses of awareness.

The internal and external focuses of awareness combine to carry into the moment a conceptual predisposition to awareness. The internal focus of awareness delimits that conceptual predisposition within the dimension of time and gives rise to the species of properties subsumed within the archetypical concept of energy. The external focus of awareness delimits that conceptual predisposition within the dimensions of space and gives rise to the species of properties subsumed within the archetypical concept of matter. The synthesis of the internal and external focuses of awareness therefore constitutes a conceptual predisposition that is bounded, or delimited, in time and space and that exhibits properties cognizable in terms of energy and matter.

Within the contemplation of the practice, the internal and external focuses of awareness are understood to represent, respectively, the intensity and specificity of focus. Both the internal intensity of the focus of awareness and the external specificity of the focus of awareness are accessible to will in the equilibrium of equal oppositions immediately prior to the moment of conceptual awareness. If will does not act, the forces of determinism entirely control the rise of conceptual awareness within the moment.

The synthesis of the forces of determinism and the force of will is governed by the requirement that conceptualization and awareness ultimately arise within the moment as a unified state of conceptual awareness. The forces of determinism (acting through conceptualization) and the force of will (acting through awareness) intersect within the present moment, where they are synthesized with one another in a process of mutual summation or diminution in the nature of wave superposition.

The internal and external focuses of awareness and conceptualization merge through superposition into a unified episode of conceptual awareness possessing unitary, synthesized internal and external focuses. Any exercise of will, therefore, alters the conceptualization that otherwise would manifest in the moment as a result of the forces of determinism. In addition, however, the conceptual disposition to awareness created by exercise of will is itself altered by its synthesis within the moment with the forces of determinism.

There is an *order of focus* within each manifestation of conceptual awareness. If the external focus to conceptual awareness manifests prior to the internal focus, conceptual awareness will arise within the present moment oriented as volition. If the internal focus to conceptual awareness manifests prior to the external focus, conceptual awareness will arise as attention. Both awareness and conceptualization carry an order of focus into the present moment. If awareness and conceptualization enter the moment oriented in an opposition of volition and attention, the stronger orientation controls the moment but is diminished in force by the magnitude of opposition. If, however, awareness and conceptualization enter the moment oriented in a unison of either volition or attention, that orientation controls the moment but with a force equal to the sum of both constituent orientations.

Volition and attention cannot simultaneously occupy the same moment of conceptual awareness. Conceptual awareness arises with singularity in one form or the other, yet these opposing aspects of conceptual awareness operate through complementary reciprocity over time. Consequently, attention and volition arise in consciousness in a dynamic balance, just as all relative dualities of equal opposition are resolved in dynamic equilibrium over time.

According to the rule of determinism, then, the realm of conceptualization is entirely controlled by the forces of determinism. There is no room within the conceptualized universe of time and space for the exercise of direct control by will. It is only outside of the framework of conceptualization, where the principle of indeterminacy governs, that will can operate as a causal agency.

Awareness, therefore, is accessible to the causal force of will only at the boundaries of conceptualization. This is *the rule of will*. The boundaries of conceptualization consist of the limitations of conceptual objects and the failures of conceptual processes within finite time and space. All conceptual objects are defined through some conceptual process. Because all conceptual processes are limited by failure, all definitions of objects in time and space are destined to end in failure. In other words, concepts are defined by their limits, and their limits are defined through the inevitable failures of the definitional processes. Will, therefore, is accessible as a causal agency only at a point of conceptual failure within any process. Such points of failure describe the boundaries of conceptualization. Within the practice, these limitations and failures are found within the present moment, where the very terms of cognition originate in the fusion of conceptualization and awareness. The willpower of the mind, therefore, becomes accessible within the present moment at the boundaries of conceptualization.

Right Practice consequently involves *the pursuit of failure* within the present moment of conceptual awareness. It is only within the realm of conceptual failure, on the borders of conceptual awareness, that the force of will is operative.

The Pursuit of Failure

> *I began again. But little by little with a different aim, no longer in order to succeed, but in order to fail. Nuance.*
>
> Samuel Beckett

The concept of failure, therefore, is central to a Theory of Right Practice. There are two meanings to the concept of failure. A particular conceptual process can terminate either in ultimate failure at its conceptual limits or in premature cessation at some point short of ultimate failure. In the absence of will, all conceptual processes will arise and vanish according to the laws of determinism. Only rarely do the forces of determinism extend a particular conceptual process to its absolute performance limits. The vast preponderance of conceptual processes subject to the unmodulated forces of determinism will terminate short of the absolute limits of those processes. Such a premature cessation of a conceptual process becomes a failure of that process only by the imposition of performance criteria that require that the process continue beyond the point of cessation. In other words, the cessation of the subject process becomes premature, and therefore a failure, only in relation to some conceptualized state of process reflecting its continuation beyond that point of cessation. Such a conceptualized state of a process is embodied in an *image of purpose*.

Within a purely deterministic cosmology, the concept of failure, like the concept of practice, is meaningless. There is only the process—the arising and cessation of process. Failure necessarily implies a missed opportunity to exercise individual will to prevent the cessation of a specific process prior to some conceptual image of purpose. In other words, there must be an opportunity for the process to continue given the right application of individual will; but equally, there must be forces operating on the process to terminate it absent such an exercise of will.

Will is meaningful, therefore, only as a divergence from the causal forces of determinism that are controlling within the realm of conceptualization. To the degree that will controls the entry of awareness into the moment, it unavoidably but indirectly will modulate the episodic manifestation of conceptual awareness, which, in the absence of will, would be wholly defined by the forces of determinism. Put differently, the concept of practice, which presupposes an exercise of the causal agency of individual will, necessarily causes some degree and respect of modulation to the causal forces of determinism.

It makes no sense to speak of the individual will of any distinguishable system if there is no departure in the behavior of that system from behavior determined entirely by the mechanistic interaction between that system, including its constituent elements, and the external universe. Each exercise of individual will, therefore, produces a departure of conceptual awareness from the systems of proportionality and probability that underpin the deterministic mechanism of conceptual cognition. Yet such departures from predictable (i.e., probable) patterns of conceptualization must occur at a level that is transcendent to the evidenciary basis for prediction, thereby avoiding disruption and consequent annihilation of the predictive framework. Such transcendence is attainable only outside the limits of time and space that circumscribe conceptualization—that is, beyond the borders of conceptual cognition.

Within the practice, the boundaries of conceptualization are found in the present moment, where time and space originate in the fusion of the forces of determinism and will. The forces of determinism operate only on and within the realm of conceptualization. The force of will operates only on and through the processes of awareness. The forces of determinism and the force of will are synthesized as they enter the moment, and this superposition of forces manifests within the moment as a hybridized state of conceptual awareness. Above all else, then, Right Practice must embrace this present moment of conceptual awareness, for it is only within the moment that the force of will can play on the failures of conceptualization.

There are therefore two potential controlling forces within each moment of conceptual awareness: determinism and will. The potential failures of the premature cessations of conceptual processes obligated by the forces of determinism are the points of vulnerability to the force of will acting through awareness. Right Practice involves the application of the force of will to extend a particular conceptual process beyond the potential failure obligated by the forces of determinism in pursuit of the image of purpose in terms of which the cessation of process became a failure of process. Right Practice therefore will consist of the progressive extension of the subject process in the direction of absolute systemic failure. And consummate Right Practice will involve an image of purpose that contemplates absolute systemic failure.

Right Practice therefore involves the formulation of a purpose that will serve to direct and control the exercise of the force of will. The purpose that is formulated, of course, exists as a state of conceptual awareness. Purpose, like any other concept, arises within the present moment as a synthesis of awareness and conceptualization. Once formulated in conceptual awareness, an image of purpose can act upon both awareness and conceptualization prior to subsequent moments of conceptual awareness. As a conceptualization, the image of purpose is fully insinuated into the deterministic realm of conceptualization. As bare awareness, though, the image of purpose remains subject to the force of will within the indeterminate realm of awareness. The concept of purpose, therefore, can be mobilized to influence both the force of will and the forces of determinism. It is this initial formulation of an image of purpose through the force of will that distinguishes practice from mere experience.

Because the will exists only outside the temporal and spatial boundaries of conceptual awareness and is therefore essentially undefinable and unanalyzable, the only test for its existence and nature is entirely subjective. It is upon some abstract precognitive and absolutely subjective level, then, that an individual can sense and control the operation of the will to shape the conceptual awareness that arises within the moment. From this subjective level of faith and belief, the force of will has the capacity to act directly to shape each successive present moment of conceptual awareness. And by shaping conceptual awareness as purpose—whether manifest as volition or as attention—the will insinuates itself into the forces of determinism that influence subsequent manifestations of conceptual awareness. The force of will therefore can act within each present moment both directly through its own effect and indirectly through the forces of determinism, manifest as conceptualizations of purpose, which were shaped by the prior exercise of the willpower of the mind.

Images of purpose define the specific discipline of body or mind that is to be practiced. The image can either encompass the entire performance system as an integrated, unitary macrosystem or embrace only a specific constituent microsystem. The principle of Right Practice, taken in conjunction with its subsidiary rules, encourages both the identification of the image of purpose with maximum specificity and the pursuit of that specific image of purpose with maximum intensity.

The specification of a particular purpose prescribes certain performance criteria against which the forces of determinism can be measured. The performance limitations imposed on a performance system by the forces of determinism become failures of that system when the image of purpose contemplates performance beyond those artificial limits. In each present moment in which the forces of determinism mandate a conceptualization that fails to satisfy the performance criteria specified in the image of purpose, a *performance gap* is created. The purpose of Right Practice becomes, then, the *bridging* of this performance gap. The force of will is accessible within the present moment of awareness in order to extend the performance that otherwise would be limited by the forces of determinism in the direction of the image of purpose. Put differently, when there is a performance gap between the performance system mandated by the forces of determinism and the performance system embodied in the image of purpose, the force of will can be mobilized to bridge that gap.

The proper exercise of the willpower of the mind, therefore, involves the identification of images of purpose with maximum specificity and the subsequent pursuit of those images of purpose with maximum intensity. At each point within the practice at which the forces of determinism ordinarily would cause the practice to fail in its pursuit of the image of purpose, the force of will becomes accessible to sustain the practice in the direction of the image of purpose. In this respect, then, Right Practice can be understood to involve the pursuit of failure. Failure becomes the benchmark against which both the specificity and the intensity of practice are determined and measured. The thrust of the mind into the moment as attention permits the identification of the potential points of failure within the purposeful practice, whereas the thrust of the mind into the moment as volition permits the purposeful practice to be sustained beyond those points of potential failure.

Right Practice consequently involves a balanced and alternating application of the centripetal receptivity of *volitional awareness* and the centrifugal projectivity of *attentive awareness*. Attentive practice demands a *soft focus*, in which the mind is held gently by will in a posture of receptivity. Volitional practice requires a *hard focus*, in which the mind is held rigidly by will in a posture of projectivity. Within the practice, the force behind both the soft focus of the mind as attention and the hard focus of the mind as volition is the power of the will.

The Theory of Right Practice presented in this book is based on the proposition that acts of mind, like acts of body, involve integral processes that can be extended to their limits only through the application of the willpower of the mind. High achievement in any performance system, whether it involves acts of body or acts of mind, will not occur spontaneously as a simple product of experience as mandated by the forces of determinism. To the contrary, high achievement necessarily involves the disciplined exercise of the will to extend the processes integral to the contemplated purpose beyond the failures of those processes that otherwise would be unavoidable. The performance system to be practiced therefore must be identified with maximum specificity and pursued with maximum intensity. That pursuit must remain focused within the present moment of conceptual awareness. There, within the present moment, Right Practice confronts the forces of determinism with the willpower of the mind.

Right Practice involves, then, the pursuit of conceptual failure within the moment by force of will. It does not, however, involve acquiescence in the conceptual failures it pursues. To the contrary—and this is of cardinal importance—Right Practice seeks, through force of will, to sustain or generate processes doomed to the failures of premature cessation by the forces of determinism. Right Practice requires, therefore, that the weakest points within the forces of determinism be opposed by the strongest force of will. The strongest force of will is developed and directed through Right Practice of volitional awareness, whereas the weakest points within the forces of determinism are identified through Right Practice of attentive awareness. These weak points are the potential failures of conceptual processes and are accessible only within the present moment.

Will, through the exercise of control within the moment, potentially controls both past and future. The past exists only as conceptual memory and potentially reflects the application of awareness within successive present moments. The future exists only as a conceptual extrapolation from this conceptual memory and unfolds only as a succession of present moments. Moreover, the exercise of will to extend any particular conceptual system beyond the artificial limits imposed by the forces of determinism extends those same limits of determinism for subsequent manifestations of that same conceptual system.

The essence of Right Practice, therefore, lies in the proper exercise of will within the moment. Within a pure discipline of mind, will is invoked to turn awareness against conceptualization in an attempt to witness conceptual awareness in the moment of its arising. Buddhist Vipassana meditative practice is an example of such a pure discipline of mind. Through Right Practice of a pure discipline of mind, the agency of will is trained with maximum effect.

Formal Practice

If he wants to work on himself, he must destroy his peace. To have them both is in no way possible. A man must make a choice. But when choosing the result is very often deceit; that is to say, a man tries to deceive himself. In words he chooses work but in reality he does not want to lose his peace. Such submission is the most difficult thing there can be for a man who thinks that he is capable of deciding anything.

P.D. Ouspensky

For purposes of analysis, formal practice can be divided into two general categories: those practices emphasizing acts of mind and those emphasizing acts of body. At the outset it should be noted that this bifurcation of formal practice is approximate and, in a sense, misleading. All subjective experiences of conceptual awareness are, preliminarily and essentially, acts of mind. Nevertheless, this differentiation is illuminating.[1] In addition, formal practice involving acts of either body or mind can be distinguished in terms of whether the practice is process-oriented or product-oriented. This distinction also turns out to be somewhat equivocal, although the underlying basis for the discrimination is both real and significant. An explanation of these distinctions—that is, between acts of body and acts of mind and between process-oriented practice and product-oriented practice—follows.

The designation of a category of practice as emphasizing acts of body must be hedged by an implicit recognition that such acts of body are themselves grounded in prior acts of mind. Images of purpose that contemplate acts of body are entirely and only acts of mind. Practices emphasizing acts of body therefore are, in their most fundamental sense, systems and processes of conceptual awareness rather than systems and processes of a corporeal universe external to mind.

An analogy to the distinction between a computer and the computer's programmer is illustrative of the discrimination between acts of body and acts of mind. The body, like the computer, is a nonsentient mechanism that must be orchestrated and animated from external sources. The mind, like the programmer, is the sentient externality that gives rise to articulate responses within the nonsentient mechanism. Practice resides only within the conceptual realm of the programmer. The deterministic realm of the computer is mere process.

Within the Physiological Model of Mind and the Physiological Model of Physical Training, the neural mechanisms of motor control are conceived as consisting of a repertoire of local motor apparatuses that are potentially independent of the mechanisms of volitional awareness. Coordinated motor response, even involving extremely complex motor performance, commonly occurs through the automatic sensory-motor mechanism without an accompanying sense of awareness. It is not, therefore, the actual operations of local motor apparatuses or of the automatic sensory-motor mechanism, however sophisticated they might be, that constitute the category of practice emphasizing acts of the body. Such nonconscious operations are analogous to the mechanistic realm of the computer.

Right Practice, because it presumes the application of the force of will, can act only on and through awareness; and awareness is, in essence, an act of mind. Yet without question, the force of will acting through awareness can be utilized to "program" the body's mechanisms of motor response. Practices emphasizing acts of body, therefore, consist of systems of conceptual awareness that are designed to program a specific pattern of motor response. The observation of neurophysiologist Ragnar Granit bears reiteration: "What is volitional in voluntary movement is its purpose." Right Practice involving acts of body is properly understood to involve the conceptualization and pursuit of an image of purpose, and images of purpose are acts of mind.

The application of the principle of Right Practice to the class of practices emphasizing acts of body is exemplified within athletic training. All four general parameters of performance implicated in acts of the body—that is, endurance, strength, power, and coordination—and all the subsidiary microsystems embodied within these performance parameters can be understood to involve conceptualized processes that are artificially limited. The artificial limit in each case will involve the premature cessation of the process dictated by the forces of determinism. The enhancement of the process therefore would require the sustaining of that process, through force of will, beyond its artificial limits. Ultimately, the goal of Right Practice must be to pursue the absolute failures of physiological incapacity.

In other words, will is accessible as a causal force in those moments within the training exercise in which the forces of determinism would cause premature failure of the exercise. The premature failure of exercise inevitably will involve the premature cessation of a specific constituent (limiting) microsystem involved in the exercise. Design of Right Practice requires that the microsystem destined by the forces of determinism for premature cessation be identified with maximum specificity. Design of Right Practice further demands that performance criteria, embodied within an image of purpose, be applied that transmute the premature cessation of that microsystem into the failure of a conceptual process. A performance gap is thereby delineated with maximum specificity between the performance system subject to premature failure and the image of purpose. By employing the force of will, moment to moment, to sustain the training exercise past such points of premature microsystemic failure, the performance of that particular episode of exercise is enhanced. In addition, such attempts to bridge the performance gap through force of will trigger microsystemic adaptations that permit the forces of determinism to sustain exercise in subsequent similar episodes beyond the point of premature cessation operant within the instant episode. The more technically proficient the practitioner becomes in the achievement of each task-specific movement of body, the less need there is for conceptual awareness to be directed by force of will to control that act of body. Instead, the act becomes increasingly automatic through Right Practice, freeing conceptual awareness to be focused evermore directly on the acts of mind that define the underlying conceptual purpose.

Design of an athletic training regimen consequently must target the microsystem to be trained with maximum specificity and must designate performance criteria with respect to that microsystem that demand maximum intensity of microsystemic function. Most athletic practice will embrace some fundamental performance objective, and this objective properly will be embodied in a general image of purpose. That general image of purpose then must be broken into subsidiary images of purpose that target discrete performance objectives with maximum specificity. Each microsystem that is potentially limiting to a specific performance objective must then be trained with maximum intensity.[2]

All systems of movement—from athletics to musicianship to speech—become accessible to the force of will in moments of potential microsystemic failure. It is here, within the present moment of potential failure, that acts of body are trained. And they are trained in pursuit of the absolute microsystemic failures of physiological incapacity.

The category of practices emphasizing acts of mind includes all of the systems of conceptual awareness not directly and proximately controlling acts of body (except, perhaps, internal acts of the brain). Such acts of mind have no discernible behavioral aspect. Indeed, from the perspective of the ascendancy of mind, they can be understood to have no direct material aspect at all and to exist exclusively within the realm of abstraction. To the degree that acts of mind give rise to acts of body, they do so on a level once or twice removed, operating either through practices emphasizing acts of body or through automatic motor response. The practices emphasizing acts of mind characteristically arise as the various processes of thought, including knowledge, understanding, logic, reason, intellect, belief, imagination, creativity, and ideation. In all cases, practices of mind arise as conceptual awareness.

Practices emphasizing acts of mind begin with the conceptualization of an image of purpose. That purposefulness is readily apparent in practices emphasizing acts of body. In a sense, the very purpose of controlling motor response through conceptual awareness embodies an object or product to which such practices are directly tethered. Because their object or goal is palpable and material, involving as they do the manifestation of human behavior, practices emphasizing acts of body are easily understood as purposeful. Practices emphasizing acts of mind, however, by definition lack such an evident and corporeal object in which to manifest. Still, practices of mind must be oriented and directed with respect to some conceptual purpose. For practices of mind, though, unlike practices of body, the image of purpose remains sequestered in the incorporeal realm of conceptualization. In other words, the achievement of the image of purpose underlying practices of mind manifests in the incorporeal realm of conceptual awareness, whereas the achievement of the image of purpose underlying practices of body manifests in the corporeal universe of physical behavior.

The application of the principle of Right Practice to acts of mind therefore is more abstract, though no less direct, than its application to acts of body. The four general conceptual parameters implicated in acts of mind—that is, matter, energy, space, and time—and all subsidiary conceptual microsystems integral to these parameters involve conceptual processes, or chains of awareness, that are limited. The limit in each case involves the premature cessation of the chain of awareness. The enhancement of a particular conceptual process therefore requires that it be sustained by force of will beyond the episodic limits dictated by the forces of determinism. Ultimately, the goal of Right Practice must be to pursue the absolute failures of conceptual incapacity.

The processes of mind involve associations and differentiations between conceptual objects and processes. The development of a complex idea through sophisticated systems of reasoning, for example, involves processes of association and differentiation that subject conceptual objects to the operations of conceptual processes. A conceptual system of association or differentiation between concepts involves a chain of conceptual awareness that can be sustained through successive present moments by either the forces of determinism or the synthesized forces of determinism and will. Just as every physical system terminates eventually in absolute systemic failure, so too does every system of conceptual awareness terminate ultimately in absolute failure. The forces of determinism, however, tend to obligate premature cessation of a conceptual system—that is, the termination of the conceptual process, or the breaking of the chain of conceptual awareness—prior to absolute systemic failure. Absolute systemic failure therefore must be pursued through force of will.

The premature cessation obligated by the forces of determinism within a particular system of conceptualization becomes a potential systemic failure that is vulnerable to the force of will only through the imposition of conceptual performance criteria that are left unsatisfied by the cessation of systemic function. Such conceptual performance criteria are embodied within a conceptual image of purpose. It is, then, the potential failures within a conceptual process, prior to absolute systemic failure, that constitute points of accessibility for the force of will. All such points, of course, are accessible only within the present moment of conceptual awareness.

Most acts of mind do not involve an image of purpose that requires that the conceptual process involved be pursued to absolute systemic failure. Indeed, when a chain of conceptual awareness is pursued to absolute failure, it departs the realm of rationality and intelligibility. Most acts of mind, however, involve the pursuit of greater rationality and intelligibility and not the pursuit of irrationality. Consequently, to the degree that specific acts of mind are product-oriented, they will eschew the irrationality of absolute systemic failure in their pursuit of rationality.[3] Nonetheless, the closer the conceptual image of purpose approaches the absolute performance capability of a particular chain of conceptual awareness, the more likely it is that a break in the conceptual chain will constitute a failure of that process. And it is within such potential failures of conceptual processes that the force of will can become controlling.

Original acts of mind, which Bohm termed unconditioned acts of intelligent perception—whether manifest as genius, creativity, penetrating insight, revelatory understanding, enlightenment, or the like—all are the product of practices involving the extension of chains of conceptual awareness, through force of will, beyond the potential conceptual failures obligated by the forces of determinism. In fact, original, creative acts of mind ultimately issue only from such a discipline of mind.

Creative acts of mind invariably involve the bridging of a conceptual gap between some prematurely broken chain of conceptual awareness and a specific conceptual image of purpose. Viewed in this way, Right Practice with respect to acts of mind involves the identification of the points of potential premature cessation of a particular chain of conceptual awareness and the recruitment of the willpower of the mind to extend that chain of conceptual awareness beyond that potential point of failure in the direction of the image of purpose. Both the point of potential failure within the chain of conceptual awareness and the image of purpose must be defined with maximum specificity. And by identifying both the chain of conceptual awareness destined to premature failure and the image of purpose with maximum specificity, the nature and extent of the conceptual gap also is defined with maximum specificity. Right Practice then requires that the willpower of the mind, manifest alternatively as attention and volition, be mobilized within the present moment of conceptual awareness in an effort to bridge the conceptual gap. Most frequently, Right Practice involves the recruitment of the force of will to extend a chain of conceptual awareness otherwise doomed to failure beyond that potential point of failure and across the conceptual gap in the direction of the image of purpose. In addition, however, Right Practice involves techniques of reverse conceptualization, in which the image of purpose is extended in a reverse direction into the conceptual gap. In effect, therefore, Right Practice involves the utilization of the willpower of the mind to bridge the conceptual gap from both directions.

Right Practice, in other words, involves the invocation of the force of will within the present moment to sustain a chain of conceptual awareness beyond the moment of potential conceptual failure obligated by the forces of determinism. Not only does the imposition of will extend the function of the instant conceptual process beyond the limits dictated by determinism, but even those limits of determinism are thereby extended for subsequent exercises of that same chain of conceptual awareness. This incremental advance along the path of Right Practice is, in essence, a discipline of mind. The eminent German philosopher Arthur Schopenhauer observed in the early 19th century that ''[t]he greatest intellectual capacities are only found in connection with a vehement and passionate will.'' Right Practice requires that the will must be not only vehement and passionate, but that it also must be disciplined.

The penultimate practice of mind is a pure discipline of mind. Within a pure discipline of mind, the force of will is utilized to focus awareness on conceptualization within each moment, thereby enabling the mind to witness conceptual awareness in the moment of its arising.

Few individuals, especially within the West, perceive sufficient relevancy to the practice of a pure discipline of mind to inspire and sustain the relentless, interminable rigor of effort it demands. Indeed, the very identification of some relevancy to pure practice implies a product orientation that potentially compromises the purity. For the vast majority of humanity, therefore, a discipline of mind becomes meaningful only insofar as it can be utilized to enhance or inform practices that are, at least to some degree, product-oriented.

A pure discipline of mind cannot be product-oriented. Ultimate knowledge is not accessible as an objectified product that can exist separate and apart from the practice. Even the state of illumination and enlightenment that is the goal of Eastern mental practice is accessible only within the actual practice. Enlightenment is not an object or product that exists in any discernible configuration of matter and energy in space and time apart from the actual experience of practice.[4] The penultimate image of purpose, in other words, becomes the pursuit of Right Practice itself.

Pared to its most fundamental essence, then, Right Practice does not pursue separate states or products; rather, it pursues only itself. Moreover, to the degree that a product orientation intrudes within actual practice, the efficacy of that practice is to some degree compromised. The primary reason for this defilement of the discipline of practice by a product orientation is simple. Right Practice involves, preeminently, the pursuit of awareness within the present moment; and a product orientation deflects awareness from the moment into a conceptual future extrapolated from a conceptual past.

There is, as well, a second, less emphatic sense in which pure practice is corrupted by a product orientation. Right Practice seeks, through force of will, to sustain or generate processes beyond points of premature failure obligated by the forces of determinism. Right Practice therefore involves the imposition of performance criteria that are designed to extend the specific process beyond the performance limit that would be mandated by the forces of determinism. A product orientation to practice, however, potentially imposes performance criteria that reflect considerations entirely unrelated to the performance limits compelled by the forces of determinism. Such product-oriented performance criteria—as, for example, victory in competition against other individuals—may or may not require that the processes involved be pursued through force of will beyond the limits of premature failure obligated by the forces of determinism.

The distinction between product and process is, of course, somewhat ambiguous. This ambiguity becomes paramount with respect to the design of a future system of practice. Put simply, a future process orientation, conceived in the design of a practice, is also a product. All future processes, in other words, are also conceptual products until they are engaged in practice by the practitioner. Consequently, the distinction must be recognized between actual present practice, or formal practice, and the design of a future practice. During formal practice, the distinction between a process orientation and a product orientation is relatively unambiguous; that is, conceptual awareness must be focused on processes that are integral to the performance system being practiced rather than on some extraneous product. Within formal practice, the image of purpose must be process-oriented. The design of a future practice, however, inevitably will involve some degree of product orientation.

The distinction between process and product in the design of a practice therefore turns on whether the product orientation of a particular design of practice will become a process orientation during formal practice. In athletics, for example, the product orientation of a tournament purse will not become a process orientation during tournament play. This is, then, a product orientation to practice. A future product orientation embodying a particular performance standard, in contrast, can be transformed during formal practice into a process orientation.

Although a design for future practice grounded in a product orientation is therefore not in itself antagonistic to Right Practice, any product orientation that arises within the formal practice unavoidably will compromise the efficacy of that practice. Practices that are inspired and directed in contemplation of some objectified end state must themselves be entirely divorced from that product orientation during execution. In other words, despite the domination of a particular system of practice by esoteric dogma, complex ritual, or even material rewards reflecting a product orientation, the actual techniques of practice employed must conform substantially to the process orientation of a pure discipline of mind. The fundamental image of purpose within a pure discipline of mind therefore must involve the pursuit of Right Practice within the present moment of conceptual awareness. The purpose of walking the path of Right Practice is not to attain some final destination but simply to progress ever further along that path.

The fact remains, however, that pure process-oriented practice is rare. A pure discipline of mind represents a consummate level of practice invariably obscured during the preliminary stages by the pervasive seductions of product orientation. Most individuals are motivated to practice only by the promise of some ego-serving, objectified result to be achieved through that practice; and the practice generally is sustained only so long as the practitioner perceives progress in pursuit of such results. Systems of practice that are emphatically product-oriented, therefore, are vastly more common than are systems exhibiting substantial purity of practice.

The potential for incorporation of the process orientation of pure practice within the product orientation of common human enterprise therefore rests on the distinction between present formal practice and the design of future practice. A product orientation, in other words, can be utilized in the design of future formal practice both to direct and to motivate the practice in pursuit of some objectified goal. Formal Right Practice, however, cannot countenance a product orientation but must be purely process-oriented.

This distinction is, in an absolute sense, artificial. Ultimately, formal practice cannot be strictly segregated from other acts of body and mind, including the design of future formal practice. Consequently, formal Right Practice inevitably will expand beyond the confines of any contrived perimeter, eroding even the product orientation that gave rise to the artificial distinction between formal practice and practice design. Eventually, progress in Right Practice will lead to a discipline of mind that transcends product orientation altogether and that is at all times and in all respects process-oriented. Within such a consummate discipline of mind, all life becomes formal practice.

Practices emphasizing acts of either body or mind require that the mind be controlled through the force of will. That control, to be meaningful, must be purposeful; and the purpose must possess, during formal Right Practice, a process orientation. This process orientation to the image of purpose, in turn, has two dimensions: intention and direction. In other words, the force of will acts on the mind in two ways. First, the mind must be directed. In other words, it must move through practice in a specific direction, usually toward some conceptual goal. Second, the mind must be propelled or animated to move in that direction.

Implicit within these two aspects to purposeful practice are the two operational rules informing the principle of Right Practice: the rule of specificity of practice; and the rule of intensity of practice. The specificity of practice is a function of the conceptualization of direction or objective. The intensity of practice is a function of the conceptualization of intention or determination. Right Practice involves the determined, intense pursuit of a specific direction or objective. These two aspects to Right Practice are embodied within the image of purpose.

Within the practice, then, the archetypical temporal property for each image of purpose is intensity, which ranges from high to low. Intensity, like all of its subsidiary properties, is an entirely relative concept that defines itself in terms of equal opposing divergencies from a center of dynamic equilibrium. Within the practice, the archetypical spatial property for each image of purpose is specificity, which ranges from expansive to narrow. Specificity, like all its subsidiary properties, is also an entirely relative concept that defines itself in terms of equal opposing divergencies from a center of dynamic equilibrium.

Each image of purpose therefore arises as a synthesis of spatial and temporal properties. Accordingly, each image of purpose has two dimensions: an external, spatial dimension that provides direction to the practice and an internal, temporal dimension that provides impulse to the practice. And again, these dimensions correspond to the specificity and intensity of practice, respectively. The greater the specificity and intensity of practice—that is, the more purposeful—the more effective the practice will be.

An understanding of systems of practice in terms of purpose implies a volitional bias of projectivity to the practice. This implication is potentially misleading. As already explained, Right Practice requires that the volitional and attentive aspects of conceptual awareness be balanced over time in an equilibrium of complementary reciprocity. Before volitional awareness can be mobilized to imbue conceptual awareness with a particular direction or impulse, the receptive agency of attentive awareness must be recruited by the practitioner to provide a general orientation of present position and of the available directions or objectives. Or, in the terms of analysis already employed in this book, practices involving attentive awareness are employed to identify the points of vulnerability within the forces of determinism, whereas practices involving volitional awareness exploit those vulnerabilities through the application of the force of will. Right Practice consequently involves a balanced and alternating application of volitional and attentive awareness. And, although the culmination of practices that are product-oriented ordinarily will entail the exercise of volitional awareness, the culmination of pure practice cannot occur otherwise than through the exercise of attentive awareness.

A Recapitulation: Bridging the Gap

A warrior cannot complain or regret anything. His life is an endless challenge, and challenges cannot possibly be good or bad. Challenges are simply challenges.

Don Juan, Carlos Castaneda

There are two distinguishable aspects to the Theory of Right Practice. First, the practitioner must define the purpose of the practice as a fundamental prerequisite to the design of the practice. Second, once the practice has been defined in terms of its purpose, the practitioner must execute that design.

The first of these steps to Right Practice centers on the formulation of an image of purpose with respect to acts of body or mind. This image brings purpose to the practice and constitutes the indispensable foundation for the design of a particular practice regimen. The image of purpose can be either general and encompassing in its scope, focusing on the relatively autonomous performance system involved in the particular discipline, or specific and limited in scope, focusing on some functional microsystem within the discipline. The image of purpose, in the pursuit of maximum specificity, must be analyzed and dissected into its constituent microsystems, and this requires the application of the force of will, cast both as volition and attention, within the present moment of conceptual awareness.

Once the image of purpose has been identified with specificity, it must be utilized as a performance criterion to transform the premature cessation of a particular functional microsystem into a failure of that microsystem. That is, when the premature cessation of a constituent functional microsystem integral to the image of purpose is a limiting factor in the achievement of that image of purpose, the cessation of the microsystem constitutes a failure of that system within the contemplation of the Theory of Right Practice. The failure of the functional microsystem gives rise to a performance gap between the implicated performance system and the image of purpose. The purpose of the practice is then to bridge the performance gap. The design of an appropriate practice regimen therefore must contemplate the extension of performance beyond the failures of the limiting microsystems.

The second aspect to Right Practice involves the execution of the practice design. Right Practice consists of the recruitment of the force of will, manifest alternatively as volition and attention, to extend the performance of the limiting microsystems beyond their potential points of failure in the direction of the image of purpose. This requires maximum intensity and specificity of focus within the present moment of conceptual awareness in an attempt to bridge the performance gap and attain the performance goal.

The techniques of Right Practice most frequently require that the efforts to bridge the performance gap proceed through the use of the force of will to extend the performance of the microsystem otherwise destined to premature failure. Right Practice also involves, however, the occasional use of techniques of reverse conceptualization, whereby the force of will is mobilized to extend the image of purpose in a reverse direction in an attempt to project a bridge outward from the image of purpose. Techniques of visualizing, or imaging, consummate performances and achievements are the most common examples of reverse conceptualization. Ideally, Right Practice incorporates techniques designed to bridge the performance gap from both sides.

The purpose of the practice, as reflected in a conceptual image of purpose, provides the direction and impetus to the practice. Through application of the techniques of Right Practice described in these writings, direction and impetus are translated into specificity and intensity of practice. The objective, ultimately, is the purposeful exercise of a specific functional microsystem at a level of intensity that extends that microsystem to its performance limits and consequent failure. Each such episode of Right Practice that stresses a specific microsystem to failure necessarily involves the exercise of the willpower of the mind to extend that microsystem beyond the artificial limits and premature failure otherwise imposed on it by the forces of determinism. Furthermore, each episode of practice that extends a particular functional microsystem to its limits in failure through the application of the force of will precipitates adaptations within that microsystem that extend its performance limits for subsequent episodes.

The willpower of the mind can operate only within the present moment of conceptual awareness. Yet within the present moment, the force of will, whether cast as volition or attention, has the capacity to control the functioning of the physiological systems that constitute the corporeal body, including the physiological systems localized within the brain. The force of will asserts its control over the physical body by identifying certain purposeful performance criteria embodied within an image of purpose and by acting within the present moment to extend, in the direction of that image of purpose, the limiting physiological microsystem that otherwise would be brought to premature failure by the forces of determinism. The force of will enters the moment as attention in order to identify the precise limiting microsystem with respect to the image of purpose. The force of will enters the moment as volition to extend the performance of that limiting microsystem beyond the potential systemic failure in the direction of the image of purpose. And because the willpower of the mind operates on and through those physiological processes of the brain that correspond to conceptual awareness, each exercise of the will causes organic adaptations within the brain that facilitate and enhance subsequent exercises of the will. The training of the mind to bring the force of will to the present moment of conceptual awareness constitutes a discipline of mind.

Although the physiological systems and processes of the body, including the brain, constitute the corporeal field on which the willpower of the mind and the forces of determinism play, the preeminent realm of Right Practice is the incorporeal mind. The realm of Right Practice is limited, ultimately, to the present moment of conceptual awareness. Right Practice, however, must be focused on a specific performance system or discipline. Any such performance system will arise in consciousness as a chain of conceptual awareness. In other words, the image of purpose for a particular performance system will manifest within the mind as a chain of conceptual awareness.

Chains of conceptual awareness involve links between successive present moments of conceptual awareness. These links are forged primarily through the systems of logic and rationality that are the condition of cognition. All singular episodes of conceptual awareness are themselves the products of conceptual processes of association or differentiation based on prior linked episodes of conceptual awareness. In fact, these fundamental processes of association and differentiation define the internal and external focuses of each episode of conceptual awareness. Each link in the chain of conceptual awareness underlying and defining a particular concept therefore represents a potential point of linkage between that concept and all those other concepts with which it potentially can be associated or from which it potentially can be differentiated. Conceptual objects and events are understood to relate to one another only through conceptual processes. The processes of association and differentiation, therefore, constitute the archetypical conceptual processes. The terms of differentiation and association, both for conceptual objects and events and for conceptual processes, are conceptual properties. And conceptual properties, reflecting the ultimate relativistic quality of cognition, are defined through the patterns of relationship between conceptual objects and processes. From these fundamental propositions, the principle of conceptual awareness, together with its subsidiary rules, has been extrapolated.

All chains of conceptual awareness are limited. Ultimately, they are limited by the outer boundaries of conceptualization, as reflected in the rule of limits and the rule of failure. Yet chains of conceptual awareness also can terminate in premature failure at some point prior to the limits of conceptualization. These points of premature failure in a particular chain of conceptual awareness constitute the field of Right Practice. In order to make the premature cessation of a chain of conceptual awareness accessible to the willpower of the mind, that break in the chain of conceptual awareness must be transmuted into a failure. This transformation is accomplished through the formulation of an image of purpose involving a state of conceptual awareness that exists beyond the point of cessation. In other words, the identification of an image of purpose brings to the practice specific performance criteria that can be applied to the actual or potential cessation of a particular chain of conceptual awareness to determine whether that cessation constitutes failure. If the chain of conceptual awareness is understood to have been broken prematurely, thereby leaving a conceptual gap between that chain of conceptual awareness and the image of purpose, the force of will is potentially available to extend that chain of conceptualization across the conceptual gap. Right Practice therefore involves bridging gaps of conceptual awareness that are determined to exist between a failed chain of conceptual awareness and a conceptual image of purpose.

A Discipline of Mind

> The ultimate test of what a truth means is the conduct it dictates or inspires.
>
> William James

Will is the energy of individual creation. It offers the only path to freedom from the bonds of determinism. It arises outside the limits of order, beyond the boundaries of conceptual awareness. It is accessible only within the moment of creation yet can be summoned only in the face of failure.

Ultimately, failure is death. Yet it is the birth of each moment that holds the promise of life. That promise rests, ultimately, on the faith that conceptual awareness is the preeminent reality and, consequently, that the individual spirit is fundamentally free. Will is the sole instrument through which that freedom can be expressed. Will is found waiting in the moment.

The force of will is the power of belief. When the secrets of its use have been mastered through Right Practice, all creation becomes a function of will. This, then, is the discipline of mind. It is at once the summit of achievement and a never-ending path . . . the path of Right Practice.

Notes

[1]Chapter 11 contains an application of the Theory of Right Practice to practices emphasizing both acts of body and acts of mind. Specifically, the chapter applies the Theory of Right Practice to athletic training (competitive rowing), musical training (the violin), and intellectual training (creative thought).

[2]So, for example, an athlete wishing to train for maximum speed in short sprints properly would utilize training exercises of a specificity and intensity that would pursue to failure the rate limiting aspects of the contractile and energy-producing systems involved in the movements of sprinting. Long, slow runs would have little training benefit in relation to short sprinting and might even prove counterproductive. On the other hand, a marathon runner properly would target the aerobic energy system and the endurance aspect of the contractile mechanisms for specific, intense training (see chapter 11).

[3]So, for example, the philosophy of scientific empiricism cannot countenance the presumption that the phenomenal universe is absolutely relative and observer created, for when the conceptual paradigms of quantum mechanics are pursued to that conclusion, Western rationality ends. The current pursuit by theoretical physicists of a grand unified quantum relativistic field theory involves the repeated thrusts of mind against the borders of conceptual cognition (see chapter 11).

[4]Within the Eastern systems of practice, even the objectified goal of enlightenment is understood to be a distraction that seduces the practitioner away from a single-minded commitment to pure practice. Throughout Eastern traditions of mental practice there are numerous accounts of the extraordinary powers, or *siddhis* (e.g., clairvoyance, healing, longevity, astral projection, levitation, etc.), that evolve through Right Practice. These powers, however, are not to be taken as goals or ends in themselves. Rather, they are regarded as dangerous seductions to the ego that potentially will deflect the mind from the pursuit of nonattachment and selflessness. The heart of Buddhist teachings is that "nothing is worth holding on to" (Kornfield, 1983, p. 31). Powers are not understanding. Powers are not enlightenment. Understanding and enlightenment arise only within the practice, and the practice is not a thing that can be held or possessed. It can only be practiced.

11

A Discipline of Mind: Western Applications

Once you fully apprehend the vacuity of life without struggle you
are equipped with the basic means of salvation.

Tennessee Williams

Although the Theory of Right Practice presented in this book is rooted
in concrete analysis, the theory itself is relatively recondite. Having
developed this elaborate yet abstract conceptual framework, it is now possible to demonstrate the application of this theory of learning to practices emphasizing acts of both body and mind.

Athletic Training: Competitive Rowing

The sport of rowing, like most competitive sports, embodies a clear and
explicit performance criterion. The goal to be accomplished—that is, the
predominant, general image of purpose— is the propulsion of a racing
shell for a distance of 2,000 meters (approximately 1-1/4 miles) in a
minimum elapsed time. The achievement of this image of purpose requires maximum performance from the energy, contractile, and neuronal
macrosystems implicated. The first step in the design of a training regimen
therefore requires that the various functional microsystems to be trained
be identified with maximum specificity. Consequently, each macrosystem
implicated in the image of purpose must be analyzed to determine which

of its constituent microsystems will be involved as a potential limiting factor in the pursuit of the overall image of purpose.

An elite or international-level eight-oared crew will cover a 2,000-meter race course in neutral conditions in approximately 5 minutes and 40 seconds. Because of the duration of the race, both the aerobic and the anaerobic metabolic energy systems are utilized. Pacing is accomplished not so much by a variation in the application of power through the oar as by variations in the cadence, or number of strokes per minute. Characteristically, a 2,000-meter race is segmented into three components: the start, which lasts for 1 to 1.5 minutes (approximately 500 meters); the body, which lasts 3 to 4 minutes (approximately 1,000 meters); and the sprint, which lasts 1 to 1.5 minutes (approximately 500 meters). The start is rowed at a cadence of over 40 strokes per minute, and the anaerobic energy system dominates energy supply. Not only is the intensity of exercise during the start higher than could be accommodated by the aerobic system even when that system is operating at peak efficiency, but the aerobic system takes a significant period of time to reach its peak efficiency during which period energy must be supplied substantially by the anaerobic system. Following the start, the cadence "settles" to 36 to 38 strokes per minute for the body of the race. Ideally, the body of the race is accomplished at the athletes' anaerobic thresholds. In other words, the athletes attempt to settle to a cadence during the body of the race that causes their aerobic systems to operate at maximum level but that does not cause additional acidification of the muscle cell environment through significant involvement of their anaerobic energy systems. During the last 1 to 1.5 minutes of the race, the cadence is increased to above 40 strokes per minute, and the anaerobic system increasingly supplants the aerobic system in supplying energy for the sprint. The objective, of course, is to maximize energy output over the elapsed time period for the race (i.e., for approximately 5 minutes and 40 seconds).

This race plan is by no means an absolute blueprint. Variations on this general format are not uncommon, although such modifications generally are designed to obtain a psychological rather than a physiological advantage. There is compelling evidence to suggest that the most efficient race strategy, from a physiological perspective, involves the acceleration of the aerobic system to the anaerobic threshold as quickly as possible and then the maintenance of the anaerobic threshold until the last 1.5 to 2.5 minutes of the race, at which point the anaerobic energy system is increasingly brought into play. Such a race plan is reflected in a phenomenon known as "even splits," whereby the elapsed time for each successive 500 meter segment of the 2,000 meter race is essentially equal.

In light of the unavoidable involvement of both the aerobic and anaerobic energy systems in a 2,000-meter rowing race, the rule of specificity of practice requires that an appropriate training regimen target both energy systems. Characteristically, the two systems are not trained simultaneously, although in many respects the training benefits overlap.

For a variety of reasons, including the predominant reliance on the aerobic system for energy supply during a race of almost 6 minutes in duration, training for the sport of rowing generally places a somewhat greater emphasis on the aerobic system than on the anaerobic system. Indeed, many elite level crews will train the aerobic system almost exclusively during the long off-season, which lasts for almost 9 months. As the racing season approaches, however, the training will focus increasingly on the anaerobic energy system.

At their extremes, the aerobic and anaerobic modes of training differ substantially. Basic, early-season aerobic training customarily will involve steady state training, in which the aerobic system is stressed for relatively long episodic periods, or *pieces*. This kind of training can involve either relatively low-cadence, high-intensity rows of long duration or multiple pieces of shorter duration but with little intervening rest. The critical objective in training the aerobic system is to stress that system at or near the anaerobic threshold for extended periods of time.

As the competitive season approaches, the training must begin to shift to an emphasis on anaerobic training. Anaerobic training characteristically involves short-interval, high-intensity exercise with sufficient rest between intervals to prevent terminal acidosis within the muscle environment prior to the end of the training session. Anaerobic training requires that the intensity of exercise within each exercise interval be sufficient to obligate the anaerobic energy system. Consequently, each exercise interval must exceed the anaerobic threshold. During the actual competitive season, a proper training regimen will reflect a rough balance of aerobic and anaerobic training. In general, the conceptual framework for training the energy systems to race for almost 6 minutes consists of the establishment of a solid aerobic foundation on which an anaerobic edifice can be erected.

This general approach to training is reflected in the training program for the United States national men's rowing team, presently under the direction of Kris Korzienowsky. Perhaps the most effective aspect of the national team training regimen is that it specifically targets each athlete's anaerobic threshold. Early in the off-season, approximately 9 months prior to the commencement of the racing season, physiological tests are done on each oarsman in order to determine the approximate heart rate at which the athlete's anaerobic threshold is reached. During the ensuing months, then, three training sessions per week are designed as training at or only slightly below the heart rate determined to correlate with that athlete's anaerobic threshold. Each such training session consists of approximately 45 minutes of exercise at or just below the anaerobic threshold, usually broken into intervals of medium duration (e.g., 3 intervals of 15 minutes duration). Interspersed with these three sessions per week of training at the anaerobic threshold are regeneration workouts consisting of long-duration but comparatively low- (physical) intensity training. Through periodic testing, the target heart rate determined to correlate with the athlete's anaerobic threshold is adjusted upward to reflect the progressive training benefit. Training at maximum heart rate, which of course exceeds the anaerobic threshold, does not commence until immediately before the racing season.

A particular training regimen ideally should be a direct and highly specific reflection of the underlying image of purpose. By identifying the physiological systems implicated in the achievement of that image of purpose and through an understanding of the limiting microsystems involved, an appropriate training program can be designed. Such a program will embody the rule of specificity of practice. Once a training regimen has been designed, however, it must be executed. And it is in the execution of the specific training regimen that the rule of intensity of practice becomes paramount. The efficacy of aerobic training, for example, depends primarily on the intensity of that training. Specifically, high-intensity aerobic training requires that the athlete seek his or her anaerobic threshold and maintain performance intensity as close to that threshold as possible for the duration of the exercise. A highly trained athlete is able to maintain an intensity of exercise near the anaerobic threshold until fuel stores are essentially depleted, a period that can last for several hours. Similarly, anaerobic training requires an intensity of exercise above the anaerobic threshold, and that level of intensity must be maintained in the face of the substantial distress associated with maximum cardio-respiratory function and substantial acidosis of the muscle environment. It is here, ultimately, in the crucible of training, that the Theory of Right Practice is of greatest significance. Each individual athlete, in the heat of training, must seek his or her own limits of performance. The athlete must use the willpower of the mind to identify those limits with specificity and confront them with intensity in the present moment of Right Practice.

The training of the contractile systems implicated in the sport of rowing also illustrates the rule of specificity of practice and the rule of intensity of practice. Although rowing utilizes a wide range of muscle groups within the body, those muscle groups are engaged in a relatively limited range of movement. It is therefore possible to replicate these ranges of motion within the framework of a program of weight training.

The three principal muscle groups involved in rowing, in rough order of importance, are the upper legs (principally the quadriceps and gluteus maximus), the lower back (principally the erector spinae), and the upper back and arms (principally the latissimus dorsi and triceps). Pure strength is not especially relevant to rowing. Instead, rowing emphasizes power, which is a measurement that includes both the strength and the velocity of a contraction. In sum, the objective of training must be to increase the power of each of the muscle groups involved in the stroke cycle. This objective is accomplished in the first instance through the aerobic and anaerobic training on the water. There is substantial evidence, however, that power training can be accomplished with even greater efficiency within a weight room. Indeed, weight training has become a highly developed discipline in and of itself, and many high-level athletic teams have a "strength coach" on staff to design and administer a weight-training program.

An appropriate weight-training program for rowing will target the three principal muscle groups and exercise them against resistance through approximately the same range of motion and at approximately the same velocity as those movements are articulated at race cadence in the racing shell. In the weight room, however, the resistance can be far greater than it is on the water, resulting in a necessity for far fewer repetitions to bring each muscle group to failure.

The notion of failure can assume easily quantifiable values in the weight room. Essentially, failure refers to that point of fatigue at which the muscle no longer can contract against a given resistance. Most weight-training systems specify that the resistance appropriate for a particular exercise should be sufficient to cause contractile failure within a certain number of repetitions. Systems that specify extremely limited repetitions to achieve contractile failure therefore contemplate an extremely high resistance. Conversely, of course, those systems that prescribe a greater number of repetitions contemplate a corresponding decrease in resistance. Research has demonstrated that high-resistance, low-repetition weight training is most effective in enhancing sheer strength. Accordingly, a weight-training program that involves exercise against resistance sufficient to cause terminal muscle fatigue after approximately 5 repetitions would be strength specific. As the resistance is decreased and the repetitions increase accordingly, the training shifts in the direction of power training. So, for example, weight training that involves a resistance sufficient to cause contractile failure after approximately 10 repetitions permits the exercise to be executed at a greater velocity, thereby training for power as well as strength. The greater the number of repetitions and the lesser the resistance, the more specifically the training will target the performance parameter of power rather than pure strength. Additionally, a substantial increase in the number of repetitions begins to implicate the performance parameter of endurance, with a resultant training effect on the energy systems involved.

Because rowing does not emphasize pure strength, high-resistance, low-repetition training has limited utility. In general, when the resistance becomes so high that contractile failure is achieved within fewer than 5 repetitions, the contractile velocity will be too slow to produce a beneficial training effect transferable to race conditions. In fact, the profound muscle hypertrophy that frequently accompanies such pure-strength training can interfere with contractile speed and endurance. Although there may be certain circumstances under which pure-strength training is appropriate in preparing a crew, those circumstances are quite limited. Instead, the principal focus of weight training for rowing must be to enhance the power of the various muscle groups involved in the stroke cycle. The training program, in other words, must attempt to replicate in the weight room and against maximum resistance the contractile processes that transpire at race cadence on the water. Characteristically, the weight-training programs for rowing prescribe a resistance sufficient to cause contractile failure at from 10 to 20 repetitions.

Obviously, the number of repetitions that a given muscle group will be able to accomplish against a particular resistance will depend on the initial state of fatigue of that muscle group. The preceding benchmark specifications for repetitions contemplate a fresh muscle group in its first cycle of repetitions. Subsequent cycles of repetitions within the same training session should reflect a decrease in the maximum number of repetitions that can be achieved unless the resistance is decreased during the training session. Most weight-training programs specify 3 to 5 cycles of a given exercise during a single training session. The ultimate objective, whatever the particular program, must be to stress the muscle group being trained to its physiological limits in terminal fatigue. Weight training such as this, when coupled with sufficient rest between training sessions to permit the muscle fiber to recover, will generate organic adaptations within the contractile fibers that will enhance the power of that fiber for future episodes of contraction at that particular velocity and through that particular range of motion.

Right Practice in the weight room therefore requires that the athlete target specific muscle groups for training through a specific range of motion at a specific velocity. Within the framework of the prescribed weight-training program—replete with its prescription for numbers of repetitions and cycles and levels of resistance—the athlete must train with maximum intensity.

The final performance parameter to be addressed by a training regimen for competitive rowing is that of coordination. Within the sport, this performance parameter is commonly characterized as technique. Rowing requires an integrated expression of explosive power, delicate balance, and fluid grace. The shell itself is profoundly unstable, and balance therefore becomes essential in order to provide a solid platform for the stroke cycle and to minimize disruptions to momentum.

As already indicated, the stroke cycle implicates three of the body's most dominant muscle groups. At a racing cadence of 38 strokes per minute, which will approximate the anaerobic threshold in a highly trained athlete, 1 full stroke cycle takes a little less that 1.6 seconds. During that period, the body moves from a position of extreme compaction (in which the knees are bent well in excess of 90° and the upper body is extended in such a way that the chest is practically touching the thighs) to a position of extension at the release (in which the legs are fully extended and the upper body is held in a "lay back" position of approximately 20° past perpendicular) and then back to full compaction. An eight-oared crew that averages over 200 pounds per rower therefore will have almost 1,600 pounds of body weight moving through the stroke cycle at extremely high speed and with extreme stress to both the energy and the contractile systems implicated. All of this movement, of course, takes place on the precariously balanced platform of the racing shell.

Races of 2,000 meters in length and nearly 6 minutes in duration frequently are decided by margins of inches, measured in hundredths of seconds. The margin between victory and defeat, therefore, is dependent not only on power and conditioning but also on technical proficiency within the stroke cycle. The challenge must be to maximize the efficiency of the power application within the stroke cycle, and this requires the cultivation of a technique that rigorously conserves the momentum of the racing shell and that translates all muscular effort into acceleration of that shell.

There are, of course, considerable differences of opinion as to exactly what the optimal technique might be. And it certainly is not the mission of this book to attempt a detailed elaboration of any particular theory of rowing technique. However, the point of this exercise in applying the Theory of Right Practice is to demonstrate how to make the physical training process purposeful and mindful. This involves not only the purposeful design of a training regimen for learning technique but also the description of a proper approach to the execution of that design.

The sport of rowing requires that the athlete become intimately integrated with the instruments of the discipline, which of course are the racing shell and the oar(s). Crews composed of more than one person further require that all of the occupants of the shell be merged into one organic and symbiotic unit. And indeed, it is the racing shell that unites the members of a crew into a single, synchronous system.

There is general agreement within the contemporary rowing community that the stroke cycle must be conceived as a continuous, unbroken, fluid movement. The image of purpose for technique ultimately must encompass the entire uninterrupted flow of the stroke cycle, integrating athlete(s), oar(s), and racing shell into a unified system of fluid movement. Technical deficiencies arise as disruptions to the integrated flow of the stroke cycle, and these disruptions decrease the net velocity of the racing shell. For the highly proficient technician, Right Practice can proceed in terms of an image of purpose encompassing the entire integrated system of the stroke cycle. For practitioners of lesser technical proficiency, however, the image of purpose must be segregated into discrete constituent phases, or technical microsystems. There are, essentially, four readily discernible phases to the stroke cycle:

1. The *power phase* involves the explosive and coordinated contraction of the major muscle groups of the legs, back, and arms in order to exert propulsive force in the direction of travel.
2. The *release phase* links the power phase and the recovery phase. The direction of movement of both the oar and the body is reversed, and the blade is lifted out of the water and "feathered" flat.
3. The *recovery phase* involves the relaxed, smooth, and coordinated compaction of the body, without disruption to the balance and momentum of the shell, in preparation for the next power phase.
4. The *catch phase* links the recovery phase to the power phase. The direction of movement of both the oar and the body is reversed, and the "squared" blade is dropped vertically into the water.

Each of these phases of the stroke cycle can be cast as a discrete image of purpose. The touchstone of technical proficiency, of course, is the maximization of the speed of the racing shell through the stroke cycle. It is therefore necessary to examine the dynamics of shell speed during the stroke cycle in relation to the phases of the stroke cycle just identified. Computer-assisted analysis of the variations in shell speed during the stroke cycle has revealed the following significant dynamics:

1. The minimum velocity of the racing shell tends to occur approximately 30% into the power phase of the stroke cycle.
2. The most rapid acceleration of the racing shell tends to occur during the leg drive, when the oar is describing the arc most perpendicular to the shell.
3. The maximum velocity of the racing shell tends to occur as the knees begin to rise during the recovery phase.
4. The most rapid deceleration of the racing shell tends to occur during the period immediately before and after the initiation of the power phase.

The segmentation of the stroke cycle into four constituent phases correlates in important respects with these four discernible dynamics of the racing shell during the stroke cycle. Without addressing the particularities of rowing technique, it is possible to derive certain general guidelines as to technique on the basis of the cross-correlation between the phases of the stroke cycle and the dynamics of the racing shell during each stroke cycle. The following fundamental technical themes emerge:

1. The power phase. The integrity of the power phase is wholly dependent on the pressure of the oar against the oarlock, which generates the propulsive force in the direction of travel. The objective must be to maximize that force during each power phase. Maximization of force is accomplished through instantaneous, explosive application of a coordinated contraction of legs, back, and arms. It is critical that all of these major muscle groups be exploited fully, and extensive practice will be required to achieve their proper coordination during the drive. In particular, the goal in training must be to increase the quickness of the effective connection and power application at the initiation of the power phase, thereby elevating the minimum shell velocity and achieving acceleration earlier in the power phase. In addition, the practitioner must strive to increase the integrity of the power application during the leg drive, thereby increasing both the level and the rate of shell acceleration during the critical period when the oar is moving through the perpendicular (to the shell). The oar handle should move more rapidly toward the bow than does the seat throughout the power phase in order to maximize pressure against the oarlock and minimize disruptions to momentum. Furthermore, the oar handle should continue to accelerate during the drive phase, yielding a relentlessly maximal application of power against the oarlock throughout the drive phase, even as the shell accelerates. The drive is an abandonment to power through an explosion of the hard focus of volition.

2. The release phase. The release from the water is achieved by a fluid, continuous movement of the oar handle simultaneously away from the body and in an approximately 45° angle down. The objective in training must be to minimize any disruption to balance or flow as the power phase is instantaneously transformed and reversed into the recovery phase. The moment of release is instantaneous. The oar handle does not decelerate as it approaches the chest but instead is effectively deflected down and away with minimal disruption to the balance and momentum of the shell. As the blade clears the water, it is rolled feathered.

3. The recovery phase. The recovery phase requires rigorous attention to the run of the shell in an effort not only to conserve all momentum but also to accelerate the shell by pulling it in the direction of travel beneath the athlete's seat. Relaxation, grace, fluidity, and balance must be vigilantly maintained, and optimum speed must be gently seduced from the shell. The recovery is the embodiment of grace wound tight to a center of balance. Within the recovery, the athlete must maintain the soft focus of attention: poised, balanced and controlled yet relaxed and profoundly

receptive. The athlete must be attuned to the dynamics of the racing shell, feeling its movements through the seat and feet and in the hands. Quietly and meticulously, the athlete must caress the speed of the shell's run away from its natural decline.

4. The catch phase. The catch phase, which is the transition between the recovery phase and the power phase, is perhaps the most critical aspect of the stroke cycle. During the final stages of the recovery phase, as the body approaches full compaction and reach, the athlete must remain loose, relaxed, and elastic while still maintaining rigorous control and balance. The catch itself requires that the blade drop vertically into the water precisely at full reach and of its own weight. The instant that the blade is fully covered, the drive phase begins explosively. In particular, the objective in training must be to minimize the deceleration of the shell immediately before and after the initiation of the power phase by increasing the speed and fluidity around the "catch" turn while assuring that no sternward pressure is exerted against the footboards until the blade is fully buried in the water.

The preceding analysis describes only the most general dimensions of rowing technique. Naturally, the stroke cycle embodies a universe of technical subtleties and particularities that are well beyond the scope of this brief treatment. Nonetheless, it should be amply clear that the stroke cycle is sufficiently complex and multidimensional to render its mastery both difficult and rare. The four phases of the stroke cycle, together with all of the linked elements that constitute each phase, transpire within less than 1.6 seconds at racing cadence. During the start and sprint, the complete stroke cycle can take as little as 1.25 seconds. Within such an abbreviated time frame, it is impossible to make conscious and sequential applications of the foregoing technical guidelines. The stroke cycle must become, ultimately, an athletic rather than a cerebral statement. It is both unavoidable and desirable that the actions and reactions of the stroke cycle will be an expression of habit—of automatic sensory-motor patterning— particularly as fatigue increases during a race. Consequently, it is critical to develop the integrity of the technical habits.

The Theory of Right Practice provides an extremely effective system for habitualizing technical excellence. Quite simply, the automatic sensory-motor system must be programmed through the application of the willpower of the mind within the present moment of the practice. The force of the will comes to the practice in the form of attention in order to assess the limitations within the performance parameters of technique. The force of will comes to the practice in the form of volition to extend technical deficiencies in the direction of technical proficiency. And, as in all applications of the principle of Right Practice, the degree of specificity and intensity with which the force of will enters the present moment of practice determines the efficacy of that practice. For all but the most proficient practitioners, the focus of attention and volition must be on one of the four phases of the stroke cycle or on some even more specific functional microsystem within the image of purpose for technique. The most competent technicians, however, can focus the force of will on the unified flow of the stroke cycle. For these few who approach the summit of technical proficiency, the image of purpose will become the integrated unity of athlete, oar, and racing shell, and failures of technique will manifest as disruptions to the flow of both the stroke cycle and the racing shell. Ultimately, it is through the identification of potential points of technical failure through the soft focus of attention—and the recruitment of the force of will to command technical proficiency where technical failure otherwise would manifest—that rowing technique is perfected.

Musical Training: The Violin

The Theory of Right Practice also, of course, can be applied to the training of extremely fine and subtle motor skills. This is not to suggest that competitive sports such as rowing do not involve fine motor skills. However, it is the gross movements of the major muscle groups that are the principal ingredients of most competitive athletics, including rowing. To be sure, the subtleties always will become increasingly critical as the quality of performance improves. Yet for many complex motor activities, the fine motor skills are of predominant importance at all levels of performance. It is illuminating, therefore, to look briefly at the application of the Theory of Right Practice to a system of training that targets the fine muscle groups principally. Such systems of training are prominent within the disciplines of instrumental music. One of the most coherent and well-conceived of such systems of training is the approach developed by the legendary violinist and teacher Yehudi Menuhin.

Menuhin's approach to learning the violin begins with the view of the violinist and the instrument as a single, integrated system. He emphasizes the interdependence not only of the violinist and violin but also of all parts of the violinist's body, beginning with the toes and soles of the feet and extending ultimately into the fingertips. He views the commitment to the music as necessarily involving every part of the body and seeks for ''a sense of the organic whole, a readiness to vibrate, a readiness to accept, a readiness to have faith in the motion—to support it, to believe it, to accept it'' (Menuhin, 1986, p. 137). The fundamental theme of Menuhin's approach to the violin rests on this notion of faith. It is faith in the vibratory motions of the music and faith in the motions of the violin and violinist that create that music. Through this faith, the violinist surrenders to the motions and is transported with those motions to the heights of musical achievement. Right Practice, within Menuhin's system of musical training, therefore requires perfection of the "trajectories along which the motion flows."

The perfection of the trajectories of motion involved in mastery of the violin obviously requires first that the proper trajectories be known. And on this point, Menuhin is emphatic. The practitioner must have in the "mind's eye" a clear image of the perfect motion of the unified system of violin and violinist, and in the "mind's ear" the practitioner must possess a clear idea of the perfect sound and the perfect rhythm. The violinist must maintain, in other words, a specific image of purpose that embodies the vibratory motion of the music and the motions of the physical system that creates that music.

The image of purpose joins musician and music "in one even flow of body, mind, will and imagination in which everything is correct and continuous" (Menuhin, 1986, p. 125). The practice is a relentless and endless pursuit of this ideal unity of uninterrupted flow. In fact, it is precisely the interruptions in flow and unity that Menuhin identifies as the proper focuses for practice. And it is here, at the heart of the daily practice, that the integrated unity of violinist, violin, and music must be broken into certain primary functional microsystems. Through a focus within the practice on conformity with the image of purpose for each constituent microsystem, the practice can be focused with maximum specificity and intensity.

Although it is unnecessary to describe in great detail the functional microsystems delineated by Menuhin within his system of practice, a general view of those microsystems is extremely instructive. Menuhin's system of training begins by addressing separately the motions of the bowing arm and hand (the right hand) and the fingering arm and hand (the left hand). This independent focus on either the right or the left hand is further segmented into focuses on the microsystems that constitute the joints within each arm and hand. Specifically, Menuhin's system of practice distinguishes between the motions of the fingers, wrist, elbow, and shoulder. It bears reiteration that all of these integral microsystems must be coordinated into a single, organic system encompassing the entire body and instrument. However, deficiencies in technique invariably will manifest as interruptions to that integrated system, and the various microsystems identified by Menuhin represent the potential points of disruption to the ideal integrated flow of musician, instrument, and music.

Once Menuhin has segregated these various functional microsystems that comprise the functional macrosystems of the right and left hands, he describes the various trajectories of motion within each microsystem. Specifically, Menuhin describes horizontal, vertical, circular, and elliptical movements. Technique is dissected into these fragmented archetypical components to facilitate the objective of providing a conceptual framework within which technical deficiencies can be effectively addressed. They are not intended as a description of consummate technique. Instead, they are provided as touchstones of technique, which the practitioner may use in order to assess the point of technical failure and then to extend the limits of technique beyond that point of failure.

As the violinist becomes more proficient, the points of failure will tend more frequently to involve the coordination *between* these constituent microsystems. So, for example, technical deficiencies involved in what Menuhin identifies as the three basic motions of the left hand—that is, shifting, vibrato, and trill—all are fundamentally and inextricably integrated with the flexion of the elbow joint. Furthermore, Menuhin emphasizes the sequence of "active motivation" and "relaxation" within both the left and the right hands, which he describes as "subtle and delicate sensations." These and other such subtleties are the essence of technique, and Menuhin emphasizes that "it is sensitivity to and perfection of the smallest details which counts" (Menuhin, 1986, p. 100).

Right Practice for the violinist therefore consists as much in intense attentive awareness as it does in volition. The musician must recruit the willpower of the mind to maintain a soft focus of attentive awareness within the present moment of practice. That focus must be of maximum specificity and intensity. Once technical deficiencies are perceived in terms of the image of purpose, the force of will must be invoked to bring volitional awareness to the present moment of practice in a rigorous effort to cure the perceived technical failure. And, of course, that hard focus of volitional awareness also must have maximum specificity and intensity.

Menuhin's system of practice rests, ultimately, on a basic faith that mindful practice does indeed produce progress. He quotes a Chinese saying that "habit begins as a spider's thread and ends up as a steel cable" (Menuhin, 1986, p. 124). Yet there is, within Menuhin's conception of Right Practice, an express appreciation for the important distinction between determination and concentration. Concentration, which focuses the practice within the present moment of conceptual awareness, must be complete. It is the "will to continue, the patience and the faith," that lead eventually to the mastery of the powers of concentration. Concentration becomes the musician's incorporeal instrument, whether manifest as attentive awareness or volitional awareness, and it is the mastery of that instrument that is essential to Right Practice. Ultimately, the instrument of concentration must be played by the force of will, and it is trained through a discipline of mind. This is the faith that Menuhin identifies as the heart of his system of practice. Menuhin's philosophy is perhaps best reflected in his own words, which carry the cryptic power of a Zen koan: "The aim is to achieve wisdom and action with ease. That is not easy but it is possible" (p. 146).

Intellectual Training: Creative Thought

Within the objectivist and positivist traditions of the West, a particular mode of creative thinking has evolved. This system of knowledge has come to be known as the scientific method, and it is commonly understood to be the foundation for the vast and manifold constructs of scientific empiricism. The scientific method, therefore, is an appropriate vehicle for demonstrating the application of the Theory of Right Practice to acts of mind.

Although there is no universally accepted definition of the scientific method, there is a general consensus as to its principal aspects. Taken in its broadest and most unobjectionable form, the scientific method is understood to consist of a number of distinguishable stages of thought: (a) the identification of a problem; (b) the accumulation of information relevant to the identified problem; (c) the formulation of a hypothesis suggesting a solution to the identified problem; (d) the extrapolation of the consequents of the hypothesized solution to the identified problem; and (e) the conduct of observation and experimentation to test the consequents associated with the hypothesis. Although there may be disagreement as to the precise characterization of each stage of the scientific method, these five steps appear to be common to virtually all processes of creative thought. A sequential discussion of these steps follows.

The identification of a problem is the logical first step in the process of creative thought. There are, of course, numerous historical instances in which solutions have accidentally presented themselves to problems that previously had not been identified or targeted for solution. Such fortuitous occurrences fall within the category of experience-based learning rather than practice-based learning. Serendipity is not Right Practice.

The identification of a problem, within the context of the Theory of Right Practice, has two principal dimensions. First, the existence of a problem necessarily involves the premature cessation of a particular chain of conceptual awareness. Second, the identification of a problem requires the formulation of a conceptual image of purpose that is not adequately linked to a supporting chain of conceptual awareness. The conceptual image of purpose embodies performance criteria through which the premature cessation of a chain of conceptual awareness becomes a failure of that chain. The problem arises as a conceptual gap between the image of purpose and an appropriate "broken" chain of conceptual awareness. The willpower of the mind, acting through both volitional and attentive awareness, must be utilized with maximum intensity in order to define the parameters of the problem with maximum specificity. After identifying the problem, the purpose of the practice becomes the solution of that problem. Within the metaphorical terms of the Theory of Right Practice, therefore, the purpose of the practice becomes the bridging of the conceptual gap.

The second step in the scientific method requires the accumulation of information relevant to the solution of the problem. The objectivist bias of Western science mandates that relevant data be gathered by processes of observation, measurement, and experimentation. This stage of analysis frequently proves to be the most critical within the processes of thought. The reservoir of information relevant to the identified problem naturally becomes the source for components of the solution. New solutions are nothing more than the reordering of old information.

A discrete piece of relevant information necessarily will itself embody a chain of conceptual awareness. All conceptual objects (as noted earlier) exist only as associations with or differentiations from other conceptual objects. Conceptual properties constitute the terms of association or differentiation. Any relevant datum, therefore, will consist of a chain of conceptual awareness involving conceptual processes of differentiation and association between conceptual objects or processes in terms of conceptual properties. A single cohesive and relatively autonomous chain of conceptual awareness may therefore arise within the present moment as a single episode of conceptual awareness, symbolized by a particular concept. These compounded concepts, embodying composite episodes of conceptual awareness, then become potential components in further chains of conceptual awareness that potentially give rise to further conceptual consolidations within the present moment of conceptual awareness. This process of compounding chains of conceptual awareness through multiple levels of thought gives rise to the entire field of cognition and system of knowledge for any given individual. It is obviously critical, therefore, that the field of cognition be properly seeded and cultivated. This is a lifelong process, and it is precisely the focus of the theory of learning set forth in this book.

When a specific problem has been identified, it is then imperative that the individual's reservoir of information relevant to the solution of that problem be as extensive as possible. It is not surprising, therefore, that the first step to solving a problem is the gathering of relevant information. Each relevant datum, in other words, constitutes a discrete episode of conceptual awareness that is potentially available as a link in the chain of conceptual awareness that must be fabricated in order to bridge the specified conceptual gap.

It is essential that each datum identified as relevant to the solution of the problem be analyzed to assess its own internal integrity. In other words, each primary datum potentially to be utilized as a building block to bridge the conceptual gap must be examined to determine its internal cogency. This is simply a deeper level of analysis with respect to the determination of precisely where the potential points of failure are within a relevant chain of conceptual awareness. Although a chain of conceptual awareness might superficially appear to be limited at some extremely compounded level, closer scrutiny might reveal that this high level limitation was the inevitable result of an undetected weakness or break in the chain of awareness at a much earlier, less compounded level. And as with any chain, a chain of conceptual awareness is only as strong as its weakest link. In order to assure the internal structural integrity of all the concepts relevant to a solution of the identified problem, the chains of conceptual awareness symbolized by and embodied in those concepts must be analyzed with great specificity and intensity.

The objective to be achieved through the second stage of the scientific method is the accumulation and validation of all available relevant information. The relevant data must be understood and manageable not only on the most compounded level possible without sacrificing internal structural integrity but also in terms of the less compounded, subsidiary chains of conceptual awareness that are embodied within each relevant datum. This reservoir of information then will provide an assemblage of flexible conceptual building blocks available for exploitation during the third phase of the scientific method, which involves the formulation of a hypothesis for solving the identified problem.

The scientific method climaxes with the third and pivotal stage of creative thought. Following the identification of a specific problem and the accumulation of all information potentially relevant to the solution of that problem, a hypothesis must be formulated to solve the identified problem. It is here that the Theory of Right Practice is most directly applicable.

The first stage of the scientific method, through which a specific problem is identified, involves the recognition of a conceptual gap between a specific conceptual image of purpose and any adequate supporting chain of conceptual awareness. For some problems, there is only a single chain of conceptual awareness that potentially could be extended across the conceptual gap to link with the image of purpose. For other problems, however, there can be any number of chains of conceptual awareness that potentially might be linked to the image of purpose across the conceptual gap. When there are multiple failed chains of conceptual awareness terminating at the conceptual gap, Right Practice requires that these chains be ranked in terms of their relative likelihood of eventually being linked with the image of purpose across the conceptual gap. This process of discrimination and ranking is an extension of the second stage of the scientific method, which involves the accumulation and rigorous analysis of all available relevant information. Right Practice contemplates the recruitment of the willpower of the mind, manifest both as volitional awareness and attentive awareness, in order to define the limits of each chain of conceptual awareness relevant to the solution of the perceived problem. Once the alternative chains of conceptual awareness have been ranked as to their potential for extension across the conceptual gap, these chains of conceptual awareness must be subjected to the techniques of Right Practice in sequence of rank.

The essence of the Theory of Right Practice is reflected in its application to the process of bridging a specific conceptual gap. In a very real sense, Right Practice involves intense and specific thinking "around" a problem. The force of will must be employed not only to extend the chain of conceptual awareness otherwise doomed to failure in the direction of the image of purpose but also to extend the image of purpose in the direction of the chain of conceptual awareness. Ideally, the conceptual gap will have been defined with sufficient specificity that it can be bridged without too great a compounding of conceptualization. When the conceptual gap is defined with maximum specificity, it will be sufficiently narrow that it may be bridged by the addition of a single conceptual link in the failed chain of conceptual awareness. Right Practice, then, also can involve the attempt to insert an appropriate conceptual link into the conceptual gap. The wider the conceptual gap, of course, the more difficult it will be to construct a serviceable conceptual bridge. Yet through consistent Right Practice, involving the application of the force of will with specificity and intensity, the likelihood of hypothesizing a solution to the identified problem will be maximized.

Once a conceptual bridge across the conceptual gap has been formulated, that hypothesis must be compared to all alternative bridges. Analysis, therefore, cannot terminate with the formulation of a workable hypothesis but must continue until the particular conceptual bridge has been determined to be preferable to all other potential conceptual bridges. And once the determination has been made that the specific hypothesis is the best available, it then must be examined rigorously in order to determine all of its consequents. In other words, the conceptual bridge must be scrutinized in order to determine all of its conceptual ramifications. This is the essence of the fourth stage of the scientific method, in which the hypothesis is analyzed to determine its full significance, including especially its significance beyond its purported solution of the identified problem. Although the hypothesis formulated in the third stage of the scientific method is understood to link a specific chain of conceptual awareness to a specific image of purpose, the inquiry in the fourth stage is how that conceptual link and the newly forged chain of conceptual awareness might fit into other chains of conceptual awareness.

Right Practice again can be employed to maximize the efficacy of this inquiry. The hypothesis itself can be isolated as a discrete episode of conceptual awareness. As such, it is the embodiment of certain compounded chains of conceptual awareness. The appropriateness of the hypothesis as a conceptual bridge across the conceptual gap identified as the problem in the first stage of the scientific method is a product of linkages between its own constituent chains of conceptual awareness and both the previously failed chain of conceptual awareness and the image of purpose. The constituent chains of conceptual awareness embodied within the hypothesis, however, also potentially can be linked with other chains of conceptual awareness not implicated in the identified problem or its attempted solution.

The willpower of the mind, therefore, can be utilized to identify the constituent chains of conceptual awareness embodied within the hypothesis and to extend those chains of awareness in all potential directions. Once again, Right Practice involves the recruitment of the force of will, cast alternatively as volitional awareness and attentive awareness, to identify and extend, with maximum specificity and intensity, the chains of awareness encompassed within the hypothesis. Through this application of the techniques of Right Practice, the consequents of the hypothesis formulated to bridge the conceptual gap can be identified.

The final phase of the scientific method involves the testing of the hypothesis through observation and experimentation. Such observation and experimentation must be focused not only on the integrity of the hypothesis as a conceptual bridge between the previously failed chain of conceptual awareness and the image of purpose but also on the validity of the consequents that are conceptually linked to that hypothesis. This fifth stage of the scientific method involves processes of observation, measurement, and experimentation that are virtually identical to those that form the basis for the second stage. However, the fifth stage places a much greater emphasis on experimentation.

Experimentation involves the intentional disturbance of a particular functional microsystem or process. The underlying assumption, of course, is that the intrusion into a relatively autonomous physical system by an extraneous force will cause a discernible and measurable change in that system and that these changes provide information with respect to the nature or properties of that system. It is critical, therefore, that both the system subject to experimentation and the experimental force introduced into that system be identified with maximum specificity. The process of analysis that must precede the design of an experiment therefore is an appropriate focus for techniques of Right Practice. Ultimately, each of the processes of observation, measurement, and experimentation can be enhanced by the proper application of the Theory of Right Practice. Some of the more obvious applications of Right Practice to such processes have been discussed above with respect to the second stage of the scientific method, which involves the accumulation of information relevant to the solution of the identified problem.

The application of techniques of Right Practice to creative acts of mind is reflected in virtually every high intellectual achievement. One such achievement, discussed in some detail in chapters 6 and 7, was the development of the theory of quantum mechanics. Now that the Theory of Right Practice has been expounded fully, it is illuminating to retrace briefly certain of the major milestones in the development of quantum mechanics. This review not only will confirm the validity of John Dewey's observation that "[e]very great advance in science has issued from a new audacity of imagination," but it also will demonstrate the indispensable role of willpower as the engine of imagination.

One of the early, crucial theoretical breakthroughs in the development of the theory of quantum mechanics was achieved by Niels Bohr. The problem that Bohr identified was the absence of an explanatory hypothesis connecting the atomic spectral patterns observed experimentally with Rutherford's planetary model of the atomic universe. The challenge, in other words, was to formulate a hypothesis integrating the mathematical formulations of the spectral patterns of atomic elements into a conceptual model of atomic structure in which negatively charged electrons were conceived to circle a positively charged nucleus. The primary link that Bohr utilized to bridge the conceptual gap between the available experimental evidence and his image of purpose was Planck's theory of the quantum. Bohr hypothesized a planetary model of atomic structure in which electrons were conceived to circle the nucleus at specific energy levels and only to move between those energy levels in instantaneous "quantum" jumps. The spectral patterns, therefore, were hypothesized to be reflections of the energy quanta emitted when an electron moved from a larger to a smaller orbit. On the basis of this theoretical model, Bohr formulated a quantitative equation that was precisely equivalent to the equation that previously had been formulated as a description of the atomic spectral patterns.

Bohr's theoretical triumph, however, proved to be short-lived. Continued experimentation soon revealed that certain experimental protocols gave rise to twice the number of spectral lines as Bohr's mathematical formalism could accommodate. This theoretical impasse gave way before the creative intellect of Arnold Sommerfeld, who hypothesized that electrons can move in elliptical as well as circular orbits and that the axes of the elliptical orbits themselves revolve around the nucleus. Sommerfeld's hypothesis was based principally on the conceptual link of Einstein's special theory of relativity, which provided a theoretical foundation for the experimentally perceived doubling of the spectral energy lines.

Eventually, increasingly precise experimental methodologies and instrumentation revealed inadequacies even in Sommerfeld's elegant theoretical extension of Bohr's model of atomic structure. Under certain experimental conditions, the spectral patterns were perceived to be double the number accountable within Sommerfeld's conceptual hypothesis. This conceptual gap eventually was bridged by the hypothesis that the electrons also spin on their own axes in either of two directions. The phenomenon of electron spin therefore was hypothesized to account for those variations in spectral patterns that could not be accommodated within the Bohr-Sommerfeld model of the atomic universe.

Even this elaborate theory of atomic structure did not last. In 1923, Louis de Broglie suggested a radical revision of the planetary model of atomic structure. De Broglie's conceptual image of purpose consisted of a model of atomic structure that could accommodate the wave equations formulated by Maxwell to describe electromagnetic conduction. The conceptual bridge between Maxwell's wave equations and the Bohr–Sommerfeld model of atomic structure involved the conceptualization of the electron orbital as a standing wave. The electron was conceived as a particle that exists only in association with an electromagnetic wave field. De Broglie's wave relation, therefore, provided a consummate mathematical reconciliation of the quantum properties of electrons first identified by Bohr. In addition, however, de Broglie's emphasis of the wave properties associated with electrons served to underscore what had become a fundamental conceptual gap within theoretical physics. The question, quite simply, was whether elementary physical existence consisted of wave or of particle.

In 1925, Erwin Schrödinger forged a conceptual link between Maxwell's wave equations, Planck's quantum theory, and the de Broglie wave relation. The mathematical model derived by Schrödinger views elementary physical properties in terms of mathematical wave relations and is called the theory of quantum mechanics, which has since been interpreted through the formulation of conceptual bridges to various conceptual images of purpose. Among the most widely accepted of these formulations is the Copenhagen interpretation of quantum mechanics, which consists principally of the Heisenberg uncertainty principle and Bohr's principle of complementarity. As attempts are made to reach some definitive interpretation of the theory of quantum mechanics and to extend the reach of that theory even deeper into the realm of elementary physical reality, the chains of conceptual awareness begin to encounter the ultimate limitations of conceptutalization. Beyond the boundaries of conceptualization there is only the realm of indeterminacy. It is within the domain of indeterminacy that the willpower of the mind reigns supreme.

References

Bohm, D. (1983). *Wholeness and the implicate order*. Boston: ARK Paperbacks.

Bohm, D. (1984). *Causality and chance in modern physics*. Philadelphia: University of Pennsylvania Press.

Cannon, W.B. (1929). *Bodily changes in pain, horror, fear and rage: An account of recent researches into the function of emotional excitement*. New York: Appleton-Century-Crofts.

Capra, R. (1984). *The tao of physics*. New York: Bantam.

Changeux, J.-P. (1985). *Neuronal man: The biology of mind*. New York: Pantheon.

Eccles, J., & Robinson, D.N. (1984). *The wonder of being human: Our brain and our mind*. New York: Free Press.

Einstein, A. (1952). *Relativity: The special and general theory*. New York: Crown.

Evarts, E.V. (1979). Brain mechanisms of movement. In G. Piel, D. Flanagan, F. Bello, P. Morrison, J. Friedman, B.P. Hayes, P.W. Hoffman, J.B. Piel, J. Purcell, J.T. Rogers, A. Schwab Jr., J.B. Tucker, & J. Wisnovsky (Eds.), *The brain: A Scientific American book* (pp. 98-106). New York: W.H. Freeman.

Harth, E. (1982). *Windows on the mind: Reflections on the physical basis of consciousness*. New York: William Morrow.

Iyengar, B.K.S. (1977). *Light on yoga: Yoga dipka*. New York: Schocken Books.

Iyengar, B.K.S. (1981). *Light on Prāṇāyāma: The yogic art of breathing*. New York: Crossroad.

Kandel, E.R. (1979). Small systems of neurons. In G. Piel, D. Flanagan, F. Bello, P. Morrison, J. Friedman, B.P. Hayes, P.W. Hoffman, J.B. Piel, J. Purcell, J.T. Rogers, A. Schwab Jr., J.B. Tucker, & J. Wisnovsky (Eds.), *The brain: A Scientific American book* (pp. 29-38). New York: W.H. Freeman.

Kornfield, J. (1983). *Living buddhist masters*. Boulder, CO: Prajna Press.

Menuhin, Y. (1986). *The compleat violinist: Thoughts, exercises, reflections of an itinerant violinist*. New York: Summit.

Miller, J. (1983). *States of mind*. New York: Pantheon.

Nauta, W.J.H., & Feirtag, M. (1979). The organization of the brain. In G. Piel, D. Flanagan, F. Bello, P. Morrison, J. Friedman, B.P. Hayes, P.W. Hoffman, J.B. Piel, J. Purcell, J.T. Rogers, A. Schwab Jr., J.B. Tucker, & J. Wisnovsky (Eds.), *The brain: A Scientific American book* (pp. 40-53). New York: W.H. Freeman.

Pagels, H.R. (1982). *The cosmic code: Quantum physics as the language of nature*. New York: Simon & Schuster.

Patañjāli. (1953). Yoga sutras. In S. Prabhavananda, & C. Isherwood (Eds.), *How to know God: The yoga aphorisms of Patañjāli*. New York: Harper & Row.

Penfield, W. (1975). *The mystery of the mind: A critical study of the consciousness and human brain*. Princeton, NJ: Princeton University Press.

Popper, K.R. (1982). Quantum theory and the schism in physics, book III. In W.W. Bartley, III (Ed.), *Postscript to the logic of scientific discovery*. Totowa, NJ: Rowman & Littlefield.

Pribram, K.H. (1981). *Languages of the brain: Experimental paradoxes and principles in neuropsychology*. New York: Brandon House.

Restak, R.M. (1979). *The brain: The last frontier*. New York: Warner Books.

Schumacher, E.F. (1977). *A guide for the perplexed*. New York: Harper & Row.

Sperry, R.W. (1982). Forebrain commissurotomy and conscious awareness. In J. Orbach (Ed.), *Neuropsychology after Lashley: Fifty years since the publication of brain mechanisms and intelligence* (pp. 497-522). Hillsdale, NJ: Erlbaum.

Introductory Quotation Sources

Reference sources for the motivational quotations found at the beginning of each chapter and occasionally throughout the chapters are listed below. The sources are listed by chapter and in their order of appearance within the chapter. A small number of the more well known quotations are not referenced here.

CHAPTER 1

Don Juan Matus ("For me . . ."): Don Juan Matus. Quoted in C. Castaneda (1968). *The teachings of Don Juan: A Yaqui way of knowledge* (p. 11).

Albert Einstein ("The most beautiful . . ."): Albert Einstein. Quoted in L. Barnett. *The universe and Dr. Einstein*. New York: The New American Library (p. 108).

George Bernard Shaw ("Reason enslaves . . .")

Don Juan Matus ("We are perceivers . . ."): Don Juan Matus. Quoted in C. Castaneda (1984). *Tales of power*. New York: Simon & Schuster (p. 101).

CHAPTER 2

Yuri Vlasov ("At the peak . . ."): Yuri Vlasov. Quoted in R. Lipsyte (1975). *Sportsworld: An American dreamland*. New York: Pantheon (p. 280).

Yehudi Menuhin ("But strength is more . . ."): Yehudi Menuhin (1981). Introduction. In B.K.S. Iyengar, *Light on prāṇāyāma: The yogic art of breathing*. New York: Crossroad.

William Blake ("One never knows . . .")

Gautama Buddha ("Monks, when one . . ."): Buddha. Quoted in J. Kornfield (1983). *Living Buddhist masters*. Boulder, CO: Prajna Press (p. 190).

CHAPTER 3

Anonymous ("If you want . . .")

Michelangelo ("Take infinite pains . . .")

CHAPTER 4

Roger W. Sperry ("The meaning of . . ."): Roger W. Sperry (1982). Forebrain commissurotomy and conscious awareness. In J. Orbach (Ed.), *Neuropsychology after Lashley: Fifty years since the publication of brain mechanisms and intelligence.* Hillsdale, NJ: Erlbaum (p. 517).

Karl Pribram ("Not so long ago . . ."): Karl H. Pribram (1981). *Languages of the brain: Experimental paradoxes and principles in neuropsychology.* New York: Brandon House (p. 165).

Wilder Penfield ("Mind comes into . . ."): Wilder Penfield (1975). *The mystery of the mind: A critical study of consciousness and the human brain.* Princeton, NJ: Princeton University Press (p. 48).

David H. Hubel ("The mathematician . . ."): David H. Hubel (1979). The brain. In G. Piel, D. Flanagan, F. Bello, P. Morrison, J. Friedman, B.P. Hayes, P.W. Hoffman, J.B. Piel, J. Purcell, J.T. Rogers, A. Schwab, Jr., J.B. Tucker, & J. Wisnovsky (Eds.), *The brain: A Scientific American book.* New York: W.H. Freeman (p. 3).

Wilder Penfield ("Indeed, no scientist . . ."): Wilder Penfield (1975). *The mystery of the mind: A critical study of consciousness and the human brain.* Princeton, NJ: Princeton University Press.

Immanuel Kant ("But although all . . ."): Immanuel Kant (1970). In A. Zweig & R.P. Wolff (Eds.), *The essential Kant.* New York: The New American Library (p. 43).

Lyall Watson ("If the brain . . ."): Quoted in J. Hooper & D. Teresi (1986). *The 3-pound universe: The brain—From the chemistry of the mind to the new frontiers of the soul.* New York: Dell (p. 21).

CHAPTER 5

Immanuel Kant ("Thoughts without contents . . ."): Immanuel Kant (1970). In A. Zweig & R.P. Wolff (Eds.), *The essential Kant.* New York: The New American Library.

CHAPTER 6

Muriel Rukeyser ("The universe is . . .")

James Agee ("So that how it can be . . ."): James Agee & W. Evans (1972). *Let us now praise famous men.* Boston, MA: Houghton-Mifflin (p. 54).

Karl Popper ("No physical theory . . ."): K.R. Popper (1982). Quantum theory and the schism in physics, book III. In W.W. Bartley, III (Ed.), *Postscript to the logic of scientific discovery.* Totowa, NJ: Rowman & Littlefield (p. 196).

Samuel Beckett ("For the only way . . ."): Samuel Beckett. Quoted in E. Schlossberg (1973). *Einstein and Beckett: A record of an imaginary discussion with Albert Einstein and Samuel Beckett.* New York: Links Books (p. 45). From S. Beckett (1959). *Watt.* New York: Grove Press (p. 77).

CHAPTER 7

Walt Whitman ("Now understand me well . . .")

CHAPTER 8

Albert Einstein ("I believe that . . ."): Albert Einstein. Quoted in E. Schlossberg (1973). *Einstein and Beckett: A record of an imaginary discussion with Albert Einstein and Samuel Beckett.* New York: Links Books (pp. 14-15). From A. Einstein (1954). *Ideas and opinions.* New York: Bonanza (p. 342).

B.F. Skinner ("Autonomous man is . . ."): B.F Skinner (1971). *Beyond freedom and dignity.* New York: Alfred A. Knopf (pp. 200-201).

Immanuel Kant ("The will is a kind . . ."): Immanuel Kant (1970). In A. Zweig & R.P. Wolff (Eds.), *The essential Kant.* New York: The New American Library (p. 345).

Paul Brunton ("The philosophic student . . ."): Paul Brunton (1984). *The wisdom of the overself* (2nd ed. rev.). York Beach, ME: Samuel Weiser (p. 436).

Max Born ("Only two possibilities . . ."): Max Born (June, 1957). *Bulletin of the atomic scientists.*

David Bohm ("Actually, there are no . . ."): David Bohm (1983). *Wholeness and the implicate order.* Boston: ARK Paperbacks (p. 25); London, UK: Routledge & Kegan Paul.

P.D. Ouspensky ("Man is asleep . . ."): P.D. Ouspensky (1965). *In search of the miraculous: Fragments of an unknown teaching*. New York: Harcourt Brace Jovanovich.

CHAPTER 9

Lama Angarika Govinda ("The Buddhist does not . . ."): Lama A. Govinda (1974). *Foundations of Tibetan mysticism*. New York: Samuel Weiser (p. 93).

Herman Hesse ("But he learned more . . ."): Herman Hesse (1951). *Siddhartha*. New York: New Directions (p. 109).

Yehudi Menuhin ("The practice of Yoga . . ."): Yehudi Menuhin. Foreword. B.K.S. Iyengar (1977). *Light on yoga: Yoga dipka*. New York: Pantheon.

CHAPTER 10

Don Juan Matus ("Focus your attention . . ."): Don Juan Matus. Quoted in C. Castaneda (1973). *Journey to Ixtlan: The lessons of Don Juan* (p. 112).

Samuel Beckett ("I began again . . ."): Samuel Beckett. Quoted in E. Schlossberg (1973). *Einstein and Beckett: A record of an imaginary discussion with Albert Einstein and Samuel Beckett* (pp. 30-31). New York: Links Books. From S. Beckett (1958). *Malone dies*. New York: Grove Press (p. 195).

P.D. Ouspensky ("If he wants to work on . . ."): P.D. Ouspensky (1965). *In search of the miraculous: Fragments of an unknown teaching*. New York: Harcourt Brace Jovanovich.

Don Juan Matus ("A warrior cannot complain . . ."): Don Juan Matus. Quoted in C. Castaneda (1984). *Tales of power*. New York: Simon & Schuster (p. 108).

William James ("The ultimate test . . .")

CHAPTER 11

Tennessee Williams ("Once you fully . . .")

Index